The Automation of the Clinical Practice:

Lessons in Systems Management

Reginald D. Smith

A Memoir

REGINALD D. SMITH ENTERPRISES, LLC

DADEVILLE, ALABAMA

Reginald D. Smith Enterprises, LLC
64 Stoneview Summit Ct. Unit 5403
Dadeville, Alabama 36853

The Automation of the Clinical Practice: Lessons in Systems Management/
Reginald D. Smith. -- 1st ed.
ISBN: 978-0-9982618-0-5 Print Edition
ISBN: 978-0-9982618-1-2 E-Book Edition

Dedicated to Bonnie, Julie, and James,

This book might never have been written without their love and encouragement. They have stood by me through it all and given my life meaning.

To Leo F. Black, M.D.,

I am grateful for his vision, leadership, and support. They were essential for the success of what we were able to achieve.

To my colleagues,

Across all my years of work with the entities that make up Mayo Clinic, I was privileged to have opportunities to work with many individuals at all levels who were willing collaborators. Thank you.

The keynote to progress in the 20th century is system and organization, in other words, "team work."

—DR. CHARLES H. MAYO

CONTENTS

Preface

No man is an Island, entire of itself…;

—John Donne, *Meditation XVII*

My goal in writing this book was to write a history of the Automation of the Clinical Practice; however, without access to many of the historical committee and Board of Governors minutes, I did not feel that I could sufficiently document the process in detail. Alternatively I chose to develop this book as a memoir of my personal story, encapsulating my career in health care for the past thirty-five years, with the bulk of the content focused upon the twenty-four years I worked at Mayo Clinic in Jacksonville, Florida. Except for my family, friends, and colleagues at Mayo Clinic, few people will know, and even fewer remember, Reg Smith. Many will more likely remember the significant events associated with the startup of the first Mayo Clinic to operate as a medical practice outside of the state of Minnesota. For those people I wanted this book to recount what we accomplished as a team.

Systems and Procedures was a division, which served as an in-house consulting group comprised of industrial engineering, operations research, and health care administration trained individuals. The focus of the group was performance improvement of all manual and automated systems for enhanced efficiency and quality of service, and the primary reason I was hired. It remained a primary focus throughout my career at Mayo Clinic.

Mayo Clinic has always operated with a dual reporting structure: one for the physician staff, and one for the administrative and allied health staff. It prides itself on being a physician-led organization, with each of the physician chairs typically paired with a professional administrator to oversee the day-to-day operational management.

My role as an administrator was to collaborate with a physician partner for accomplishing our goals. I was the administrative leader for the work described in this memoir.

The period between 1992 and 2000 for the outpatient medical practice was largely dominated by the Automation of the Clinical Practice, when we made several significant cultural changes well ahead of many other practices for specific operational reasons. Central to all of this work and accomplishment was the collaboration of many people at many levels in the organization. I have tried to recognize many of the key individuals and their significant contributions to the success of the practice, and the lessons we learned.

Without the outstanding leadership of Dr. Leo F. Black this story might never have happened. His appointment of my physician partner in leading this major undertaking served as an essential support for the success. The leadership of Dr. John J. Mentel as the successor to my physician partner in bringing the Department of Applied Informatics to fruition brought a sense of vision for the future of technology in the medical practice. This story would be much less without these key individuals. If I did not mention specific people, it may be because I do not have permission from them to use their names.

My goal in this story is to recall the facts and to lay them out as clearly as possible. I was not privy to many senior leadership meetings or other discussions, which transpired above my administrative level

The reference to John Donne's line captures the essence of what I am trying to emphasize by writing this story. No man is an island—any success we achieved was the result of our collaboration and certainly made us more successful than if we had worked individually.

Collaboration is perhaps the single greatest ingredient contributing to the success of Mayo Clinic, not only with practicing team medicine but also with all levels of the clinical and professional staff.

Prologue

It was my good fortune to join Mayo Clinic at a very decisive time in my life. I was forty-five years old and ready for a change. I did not have a clue what was behind how I came to be recruited, but I do know how they learned about me, my work, and my interest in working there. As I look back at the experience, it was a complex, almost mystical process, which I still do not fully understand today, twenty-four years later. Mayo Clinic was a very large and complex organization when I joined the staff, and yet, once employed, it was as if I had become a member of the family.

The process began five and a half months earlier. Once it started, there were long passages of time in which there was no communication with anyone at Mayo Clinic. Interviewing once for a job is common. If you are invited back for the second interview, you begin to think your chance of getting the job looks promising, and you begin to believe that you might be offered a position. The process I experienced eventually involved three separate daylong or multi-day sessions with many interviews, weeks apart. There was no immediate communication from Mayo until I received a call to be scheduled for more interviews at a new location, with a new round of interviewers. Then a completely unexpected event occurred. Let me explain.

In 1990 I was working at the data-processing subsidiary of Adventist Health Systems Sunbelt, Inc. in Orlando, Florida. I had completed a terminal degree at the University of Florida (Doctor of Education, August 1983). In the process of working on my degree course requirements, I was doing extensive work with the then emerging technology of microcomputers, in the Department of Medical Education at Florida Hospital Medical Center. My position in the department was Assistant to the Director of Medical Education, with my work focused on the administrative aspects of the program.

The director was a board certified family physician with Doctor of Medicine (M.D.) and Doctor of Philosophy (Ph.D.) degrees.

The Family Practice Residency program was considered large, with thirty-six residents, twelve in each of the three years of the program. The department sponsored the educational programs for the residency and continuing medical education. The director and I worked well as a team. His expertise was in medicine, and my experience was in education, so our skills were complementary. During the course of my three years in the Department of Medical Education, I led the effort to get the institution accredited as a provider for Continuing Medical Education (CME). Accreditation as a provider for CME was a first for the nearly century-old institution.

A great review course for physician continuing medical education and resident training had been developed for the Apple II Plus microcomputer. This opportunity to provide computer-based education was too tempting to pass up. We were able to justify it as a cost-effective new venture for the department. One of my significant accomplishments was to bring in a personal computer for use with computer-based education in the Family Practice Residency Program. I recall sitting in the boardroom waiting to justify the purchase of the computer when the chief financial officer told those in the room not to worry. These little computers were like "toy calculators and will never amount to anything more."

The addition of that Apple II Plus fueled the use of computers for medical education, and it provided me with a platform to improve my programming skills.

First I developed a suite of applications for tracking attendance for the extensive medical education programs, transcripts, and reports that proved beneficial in gaining accreditation for the program. The applications I wrote were comprehensive and provided for pre- and posttesting for attendees at the programs, and they even computed the *point biserial correlation* for the test items.

The point biserial correlation compares the results for each question, and then correlates it to the students who perform well versus those who do not. If those who generally do well miss a test item, then it is likely to be a bad test item. This feedback is useful to the educator in development of future tests.

A program used in the residency to advise outpatients regarding their dietary habits was one of the applications I developed in collaboration with one of the faculty engaged in the residency program. The program was called *Nutrition Analysis 99,* and it won the Outstanding Scientific Exhibit at the annual meeting of the Florida Academy of Family Physicians in 1982.

The applications and innovations I had developed caught the attention of the senior administrators so that by the time my doctoral degree was awarded, I had been promoted to the director of systems management at the flagship hospital, Florida Hospital Medical Center in Orlando, Florida. As the director of the department, my team and I provided support to a management-consulting firm to study all of the areas of the hospital and to build a productivity monitoring system.

The goal of the engagement was to build a tool that would assist the managers and supervisors of each unit in managing the labor force, workload, and productivity. These measures usually related to providing reports on a weekly basis for the workload, FTEs, and overall productivity by work units. My team and I had a complete understanding about work measurement. Several of us became certified for Methods-Time-Measurement UA, which enables very detailed work requirements of a time and motion nature. My department was also responsible for monitoring the other operational statistics.

While I was the director of systems management, I managed to establish the networking of microcomputers. Orchid Technologies produced a product that would enable the members of my department to share files across the network by interconnecting our computers with coaxial cables and BNC connectors. It was effective and it was the first microcomputer network in the hospital.

In 1987 hospital management decided that while we had built a great productivity system, they needed to understand costs better. So the members of my team were all encouraged to become cost accountants, shifting focus away from productivity. Within a few months, the whole team had moved on to new employment opportunities, which did not include becoming hospital cost accountants. Given my advanced degree, experience, and qualifications, I was offered an opportunity to work with the mainframe computer systems, and in July of that year, I made the change.

The data processing shop was primarily IBM-based and used their product line exclusively. Senior management considered IBM to be a known quantity, and the suite of products provided the basis for an application suite, which consisted of patient management, billing, human resources, and accounting services (including accounts payable and receivable, general ledger, etc.). It was developed as part of a larger product line during the '70s.

The contractor/developer was futuristically named Space Age Computer Systems, Incorporated (SACS). I recall that whenever administration approached them about a new feature or report, the company manager's first response was typically, "Well, that is not part of the contract for services, so we will have to create a contract rider or addendum, and I'll get a quote for the added cost for you." The company had an exclusive contract to "control all of the computers at Florida Hospital."

My work of getting the first microcomputer into Medical Education, and then networking microcomputers, it later turned out, had been a point of contention between SACS and Adventist Health Systems.

After years of the organization being in an exclusive contract, SACS was given the required notice and terminated. In the meanwhile, Adventist Health Systems Sunbelt established a new data processing subsidiary named Sunbelt Systems Concepts Incorporated (SSCI). It was in this new subsidiary that I was offered my position.

My initial work involved acquiring knowledge of Job Control Language (JCL) and the COBOL programming language.

After a few months of getting my feet on the ground with IBM mainframe software development, and learning about moving software through the various environments to production, I was asked to apply my leadership skills to development of a new Master Patient Index system, leading a team with four other seasoned programmers. We had countless meetings with the director of patient accounts and designed a new system based on the extensive requirements of the documents we developed. It was towards the end of that first year of development that my team and I successfully completed conversions of more than one million patient registration records from the old system.

The new patient registration system was readied for implementation, users were educated on the new features, and the project was successfully on its way to implementation in production when I was called into my boss's office. A new system was being prototyped to use COBOL II, SDM II, DB2, and GDDM to build an executive information system.

They envisioned a system that would collect data nightly at Florida Hospital and the other hospitals making up Adventist Health System Sunbelt. The data would be aggregated to produce a variety of timely reports available to the senior management of each of the seventeen hospitals and the chief executive officer of the corporation. Based on my work in systems management, the leadership of SSCI wanted me to design how the executive information system would function. My knowledge of what key operational statistics the executives watched on a daily basis to assess the successful operation of their facility was key.

The use of the graphics terminal to display the information to be contained in table format or scaled graphs seemed to be the best technology. Each choice would be menu driven, with function keys to zoom the quadrant to full screen display. The reports would display the information in its various aggregations on a color graphics display terminal. The screen would be split into four vectors, one for each quadrant (upper left, upper right, lower left, and lower right). The lower left space was reserved for menu options, and the other three would be used to display graphic representations of the numeric data. For example, one screen might display hospital census, showing each day for the current thirty days, and the same thirty days of the previous year adjusted to match the day of the week, average daily census month to date, and average length of stay as a trend line.

The technology I was working with had not existed when I graduated from the University back in 1967. My career had been transformed to become more challenging and interesting. I was acquiring new technical skills and envisioning ways to do new and truly innovative things. Then, with everything going great guns, I got called into my boss's office again.

The local IBM representative had seen my work on the executive information system and had told his superiors about me. This was the first time IBM had a client who had built such a system, and as a result, they had some requests. The annual IBM Executive Summit was going to be held in Phoenix, Arizona, at the South Mountain Resort. The conference was an all-inclusive trip for CEOs, CFOs, CIOs, and other C-level employees. IBM wanted me to make an hour-long presentation at the conference regarding the system I had designed and built. IBM wanted to videotape the session too.

They planned to edit the video, add titles and music, and add the final production to the IBM library of educational materials they provided to their clients. My boss was going to introduce me in the presentation.

Immediately after my presentation to a packed room, with the video cameras rolling, a tall man approached me and introduced himself. He said, "I am very interested in the system you have described, but I just can't believe that it performs as you say it does. I am Craig Smoldt from Mayo Clinic, and I am in Florida almost every month for the board meeting of our new facility in Jacksonville. I was wondering if you would be open to letting me visit you in Orlando to see this system myself."

"Just call and let me know when you would like to see it, and I'll be happy to arrange a time to meet with you," I replied. That was my first introduction to Mayo Clinic, and it seemed that Mr. Smoldt was quite interested in my work.

About a month later, Mr. Smoldt arrived at my office in the corporate headquarters building. My office was small, just large enough for a desk, a small bookcase, and one side chair. I spent less than forty-five minutes demonstrating the system and answering questions. As he prepared to leave, he said, "This is very impressive. I would like to bring a small group down from Mayo Clinic and show them this system. Would that be possible?"

I asked him to send me a letter with the names of the individuals and their titles. I would review it with my superiors and get back with him. Within a week, I had a letter with the names of another administrator and two physician leaders, one of whom was Dr. Leo F. Black. They wanted to fly down in a corporate jet on a Friday morning and meet with me at noon to see a demonstration of the executive information system. Their plan was to return to Minnesota that same afternoon.

My office would not accommodate a group of that size, so I arranged to borrow the office of the CFO of Florida Hospital to host the group and demonstrate the system. I gave a brief overview of the system, discussed the design, and then encouraged one of the visitors to run the system himself. The physician was an older man wearing a gray suit over a white shirt with a narrow little tie. I did not know he was Dr. Leo Black. His crew-cut hair was gray too. I later learned that he had served in the Marines before attending medical school.

His face broke out in a broad smile when he saw the data with the graphic display paint each of the quadrants on the screen. The group saw all they needed to see in less than an hour, thanked me profusely for the demonstration, and departed.

It was nearly a year before I heard from Mayo Clinic again. There had been no discussion about further contact with them, despite their apparent interest in my work. I had no idea that Mayo Clinic would play a big part in my future.

In February 1990 my weekly copy of *Computerworld* arrived at work, and I spent some time reading about the rapidly emerging trends in computer technology. Towards the end of my browse through the tabloid, there was a display ad for information technology (IT) professionals at Mayo Clinic. By this time my work with the executive information system was well established. I had traveled to all of the hospitals in the Adventist Health System, delivering an IBM PC loaded and configured to demonstrate the system to the CEOs for each of the hospitals. I delivered the system, set it up, and verified the system performance. Then I taught each of the executives how to use the system.

I spoke regularly at Electronic Computing Health Oriented (ECHO), the IBM user group. Since my initial presentation in Phoenix, I had become a regular speaker on executive information systems. Despite the growth of my professional work, I was not getting any recognition for my contributions to SSCI. I decided to contact Mr. Smoldt at Mayo Clinic. He was functionally the Chief Information Officer (CIO) who had been in my office on two different occasions to watch demonstrations of the executive information system. I mailed a letter on Valentine's Day expressing my interest in a position with Mayo Clinic, but heard nothing for the next five weeks.

Late in March I got a call from Mr. Craig Smoldt. He asked if I remembered the letter I had sent. Of course I did. He asked me to contact the Human Resources (HR) Department to set up a visit to Rochester, Minnesota. I purchased a round-trip ticket and flew up on a Thursday morning and checked in to the Kahler Hotel, all paid for by Mayo Clinic. I began my first round of interviews at noon, followed by more interviews the rest of the day, ending with dinner.

Friday brought more interviews with members of the staff in Information Technology and Administration, and ended with a half hour meeting with the HR representative. I remember that afternoon vividly for two reasons: He handed me eight one hundred dollar bills as reimbursement for my flight, and it was my birthday. I was stunned to be reimbursed in cash because I never carry that much on my person, unless it is in traveler's checks. I was afraid of being mugged in the airport before I got home.

After two days of grueling interviews, I slept in on Saturday, had a big breakfast in the hotel dining room, and then drove around Rochester, snapping pictures of various houses for sale in a variety of neighborhoods. Although we had no idea if I would be offered a position, let alone relocate to Minnesota, I had promised my wife, Bonnie, that I would check out the area. I caught my flight home at noon and arrived in Orlando a few hours later. I enjoyed a belated birthday celebration that evening with my family. I was so glad to be home, but also hopeful of how my interviews had gone.

During the following weeks, I waited anxiously to learn if Mayo Clinic was still interested in me. They didn't call. I felt discouraged by the lack of feedback. I continued work during the day, and looked for job leads at night. I filed an application and résumé with Cincinnati Bell Information Systems (CBIS), which was one of the companies rapidly expanding in the local area. Cellular telephones were taking off at the time, with the trajectory of a space shuttle launch. CBIS was processing approximately 80 percent of all cellular telephone billing in the United States, and their staff was growing at a slightly slower rate but very quickly.

Although I didn't really want to work for CBIS, I was convinced that I was due for an employment change. I wasn't getting any younger. Plus I wanted to work for a company with stability and growth opportunities, a place where I could work comfortably for the rest of my professional life.

In May I received a call from Mr. Carleton Rider, the administrator at Mayo Clinic Jacksonville. He informed me that my interviews had gone very well, and he asked me to a travel to Mayo Clinic in Jacksonville for a daylong round of interviews, ending with a recruitment dinner in the evening. They offered to arrange a special orientation program for Bonnie, while I spent the day in interviews. She declined the offer to travel with me since she was the nurse/manager for the Endoscopy Unit at Florida Hospital Medical Center. Our daughter was attending college, and our son was in his junior year in high school.

I arose early on the day of the interviews and drove to Jacksonville. The morning passed quickly as I met with the various people on my schedule. The administrator and the interview team took me to lunch at the Point of View Restaurant, which sat on the edge of the southeast corner of Beach Boulevard and the Intracoastal Waterway. Sitting at a table overlooking the waterway, the canopy was still low enough that I could see the top of the four-story Davis Building. After an enjoyable lunch, we returned to the campus and I pressed on with my afternoon round of interviews.

Following the interviews, we drove out to The Lodge at Ponte Vedra Beach for the recruitment dinner. The entire staff in administration had been very cordial during my visit and interviews. With our experience in health care, systems, and information technology, there were plenty of topics of mutual interest.

Our time together passed quickly and we parted. I drove back to Orlando and returned to my routine work schedule. The telephone went silent again. After a couple of weeks, I again felt discouraged.

My application at CBIS had gotten my name to a short list of candidates. I was called in for an interview following Memorial Day. A week later, I learned that my round of interviews at CBIS had gone very well. CBIS called me back for a second interview; yet, there was no word about my second round of interviews from Mayo Clinic. At the end of the process, I was offered a position at CBIS, but I didn't want to accept it; I was still hopeful about an offer from Mayo Clinic. I asked for time to consider the offer, and they gave me until the end of the week. The compensation was attractive, but the job involved traveling around the Caribbean basin. Being away from my family would be difficult and would create more stress. I was facing a tough decision.

Friday rolled around and still nothing from Mayo Clinic. I felt like I could only make one decision: join CBIS. A little after noon, the phone rang. It was my contact from Rochester. Mayo Clinic wanted me to return to Rochester for another round of interviews.

I was being considered for a position to start a new section of Systems and Procedures for Mayo Clinic Jacksonville and St. Luke's Hospital. The two organizations would share the position, with an office and staff at both sites. Assuming everything went well, Mayo Clinic would offer me a position. (Although I was also informed that it was unusual for Mayo Clinic to bring in someone in a management position from the outside.)

While I was there, they wanted me to interview potential candidates for staffing the new unit. If I was offered the position, I would complete the first two months of work in Rochester: getting oriented, acquiring the Mayo Clinic culture, and becoming familiar with important contacts. We now refer to that as being "Mayo-nnaised!"

A week later, I traveled to Rochester and completed the remaining staff interviews, two of whom would become the first members of my staff in Jacksonville. Everything seemed to go without a hitch. When it was time to catch a cab to the airport, I was escorted to the front of the Kahler Hotel, but still I had not been offered a position. The driver put my suitcase and briefcase into the trunk. I began to panic. How would I go home and explain to my wife that everything had gone well…except Mayo Clinic had not offered me a position!

I finally turned to my host and said, "Excuse me, but I thought I was going to be offered a position as part of this trip, if everything went well."

My host acted surprised. "Hasn't anyone offered you a position?"

"No."

"I'm as surprised as you are. Well here is what we are offering…"

The offer of employment was made as I was literally getting into the cab to leave for the airport. I told my host, "I don't have to think about this offer at all. I accept."

After I was back home, he called and we made the final arrangements for my physical at Mayo Clinic Jacksonville, where I was signed on as an employee. My first day on the job was Monday, July 2, 1990. It would be a travel day, with me flying to Rochester and getting set up for the next two months.

Independence Day was looming, a holiday in the middle of my first week at work for Mayo Clinic. I would be in Rochester, and my family would be twelve hundred miles away in Orlando for the Fourth of July. Leaving my family for two months was one of the hardest things I have done, but I was so grateful for being hired by Mayo Clinic.

CHAPTER ONE

Starting Work in Rochester

Never continue in a job you don't enjoy. If you're happy in what you're doing, you'll like yourself, you'll have inner peace. And if you have that, along with physical health, you will have had more success than you could possibly have imagined.

—Johnny Carson

I arrived in Rochester, Minnesota, in the afternoon, on Monday, July 2, 1990. The Kahler Hotel served as my residence for the first week. I started my orientation at Mayo Clinic on Tuesday, July 3, at 8 a.m. in Systems and Procedures on the sixth floor of Centerplace. I was told the building was leased to Mayo Clinic, and served as an office building on the edge of the campus at the time. The weather was clear and sunny, with the city enveloped in a heat wave.

One of my first activities was to find a place to stay for the two months I would live in Rochester. I recall that on my way to check out a furnished apartment, I was waiting for a traffic light to change on the corner of West Center Street and Third Avenue N.W. by the Charlton Building. The temperature was 104 degrees, one of the hottest days I have endured since joining Mayo Clinic. A car turning the corner in front of me caused the pavement to buckle, and chunks of the concrete erupted as the car tires rolled over the hot roadway.

All of the apartments I checked to rent that afternoon had some problems. The first place had ample space but none of the necessary furnishings I needed. As I checked out each lead, it seemed a similar problem would surface. Finally I decided to rent an efficiency room at the Best Western Motel at Soldiers Field. Getting meals in the staff cafeterias at the Baldwin Building, Rochester Methodist Hospital (Eisenberg Building), or local restaurants was always an option, although the room they gave me had a kitchenette.

During the week, I was a pedestrian, but the Clinic arranged for me to have a rental car for the weekend so that I could get out and see some of the local attractions. I would pick up the car at the close of business on Friday and return it late Sunday evening or first thing Monday. The Clinic policy said that after the first three weeks, the Clinic would pay for a trip home for the weekend, or alternatively, I could use the funds to bring my spouse, Bonnie, to Rochester. Following the first three weeks, I would be able to make the trip home every other weekend.

The next day was hard. It was July 4 and the only Independence Day I can recall that I haven't been with my family. The section head invited me on a trip to his parents' farm for a barbeque. One of the analysts invited me to join her and her husband for a day of sailing. I couldn't pass up the invitation, so I spent the holiday sailing on Lake Pepin.

Lake Pepin is a portion of the Mississippi river that has been dammed to create a lake, nestled between Minnesota on the west and Wisconsin on the east. Readers of *Little House on the Prairie* series might recall that Laura Ingalls Wilder's Pa started the trip west by crossing frozen Lake Pepin with a wagon drawn by a team of oxen. The little house featured in the book is not too far away from the little town of Pepin, still located in Wisconsin on the eastern shore of the lake, but the little house in the big woods no longer has the big woods around it.

My hosts had packed a picnic lunch and drinks, and we sailed up the lake from the town of Pepin to Lake City, on the western shore. Once there, we tied up at the city marina and enjoyed lunch while the boat was not kneeled over or rocking. The sun broke through the mostly overcast sky and warmed things up after the cold winds we had encountered on the lake. It was quite a change from the previous day's furnace-like temperatures.

It was a nice day sailing, but I missed being with my wife and children terribly. I noted that I was to start work in Jacksonville the day after the next holiday, Labor Day, so I took comfort that I would be with my family when it rolled around.

Most of my time for the next two months had been prescheduled with orientations in many areas of the operations of the Clinic as an analyst in Systems and Procedures. My orientation included time in Information Technology (IT) learning about the scheduling systems, ordering, and charging systems. The manual processes were part of the orientation since the practice in Jacksonville was intended to clone the services and operations of those in Rochester. One project was to review the structure and organization of the microcomputer support area and make recommendations for future development. My schedule consisted of approximately 75 percent orientations with the remaining time working on projects, with the goal that they would be completed prior to my leaving Rochester.

The medical records systems especially held my attention. I remember being seated at a table and looking at some of the original medical records in a large leather-bound book. It was one of the journals of Dr. William James Mayo from 1889. It was written in clearly legible pencil and contained a summary note on each of the patients he had seen and treated. There were usually three or four entries per page. Each entry was numbered sequentially, and then the fly pages for the ledger contained hand-ruled columns reflecting the handwritten indices.

Each physician in the practice kept their ledger with the records for each patient seen in the practice. When a ledger was full of entries, a clerk was hired to number each entry, and then data was noted regarding the presenting symptoms, diagnosis, treatment, and outcome. This additional work paid big dividends when Dr. Will Mayo was invited to speak at medical symposiums. In preparation for his presentation, he could perform a retrospective review of his own cases and make inferences regarding the efficacy for his treatment and outcomes. Similarly, separate surgical case records were kept, providing a rich data repository, albeit manually assembled and recorded, for presentations regarding surgical procedures and outcomes.

In 1907 Dr. Henry Plummer invented the medical record still in use at the time. It transformed the record from those leather-bound books to a loose-leaf, multi-authored collection of documents that was circulated throughout the practice, with each physician contributing their information into the unit record. As one of the early partners in the practice, he called it the *dossier* medical record. The dictionary defines dossier as "a collection or file of documents on the same subject, especially a complete file containing detailed information about a person or topic."

He must have been quite challenged in getting the physicians to give up their medical records in leather-bound journals kept in their offices in favor of the circulating a single medical record for each patient. I learned about the subsequent indexing of the content of patient records. The Mayo Clinic unit medical record had played a pivotal role in retrospective research over the eighty-three years of its existence. Because of this pioneering medical record work, more retrospective clinical studies have been conducted on Olmstead County residents than any other part of the country.

That first Friday of my work in Rochester, I bought a copy of Helen B. Clapesattle's *The Doctors Mayo,* thinking that getting a more in-depth understanding of the Mayo Clinic founders would be good for beginning my work there. It turned out a rainy cold front arrived that weekend. With my family in Orlando, twelve hundred miles away, and socked in with rain, it was easy to pass the time reading. By Sunday evening, I had completed the book and felt a thorough knowledge of the founders.

The origin of the title of that book continues to impress me. The brothers were very close, to the point that they kept all of their money in a single checking account, used by both families throughout their adult lives. Their checks said simply: "The Doctors Mayo."

My orientation and work coordinated by Systems and Procedures (S&P) went very well. I established friendships with colleagues that have lasted my entire career at Mayo Clinic. Two of my colleagues in S&P at the time introduced me to a cheeseburger on one of our lunch hours that sticks in my memory to this day. The golf course at Soldiers Field had a grill that offered "Yo" Burgers in three different sizes: quarter pound, half pound, and three-quarter pound. As I recall, the quarter-pound burger was ample, and unless one was very hungry, the latter two would have equaled pure gluttony and made it very difficult to work for the rest of the day. Nevertheless the burger was awesome.

After I had settled into a routine, Bonnie and I talked about the family coming to Rochester on vacation to spend some time with me. Proud of working for Mayo Clinic, I wanted to show them my professional environment. We planned for them to travel to Minnesota in the middle of one week and to return in the middle of the next. That way we would have a weekend in Rochester to explore.

At the time, the Gonda building was not in the planning stage yet; however, they toured the Mayo, Plummer, Eisenberg, Hilton, Baldwin, Guggenheim, and Medical Sciences Research buildings. The manager of the Foundation House arranged a tour, and one afternoon we visited the Plummer House and Mayowood.

That weekend we crossed the river into Wisconsin. Both of our children were babies when the television series *Little House on the Prairie* was on prime-time network on Monday evenings, so we could not pass up the opportunity to show them the "Little House in the Big Woods." It sits outside of the small town of Pepin and has been reconstructed from the plans Pa Ingles filed with the township when it was first built. We had a wonderful time exploring.

As they were getting ready to leave for the airport, I remember giving them a pop quiz about the campus. They did quite well with my challenges to name the buildings. I tried to make it a fun distraction, because I didn't want them to leave. I knew the dreaded loneliness would return until the next time I could go home for a weekend. Their visit was a great boost to my morale, and I knew that in a few weeks, my experience in Rochester would be over, and then the new phase of my work with Mayo Clinic and St. Luke's Hospital in Jacksonville, Florida, would begin. I had no idea of the challenges I would be facing when I returned to Florida.

CHAPTER TWO

Feet on the Ground in Jacksonville

And let it be noted that there is no more delicate matter to take in hand, nor more dangerous to conduct, nor more doubtful in its success, than to set up as a leader in the introduction of changes. For he who innovates will have for his enemies all those who are well off under the existing order of things, and only the lukewarm supporters in those who might be better off under the new.

—Nicolo Machiavelli, *The Prince*

With Labor Day being a Clinic holiday, my first day on the job in Jacksonville was Tuesday, September 4, 1990. The four-story Davis Building had opened as Mayo Clinic Jacksonville to the public on October 13, 1986, and it had grown faster than the projections. The administrator who provided the first systems support had his responsibilities increased to the point that he was asked to move into a role as a full-time administrator, and he left his role in systems support. The next employee in that position experienced the same growth, to the point that she accepted an administrative position in operations, leaving the systems position open again.

Because of the rapid growth of the Clinic, the administrative support functions had run out of space. To address this need for additional space, the third floor on the south wing of the Courtyard by Marriott was leased to support operations. With the opening of my position, several rooms at the end of the corridor on the second floor of the south wing were leased to provide space for administrative services and Systems and Procedures, and my first office at Mayo Clinic was in this set of rooms. At St. Luke's Hospital, an empty suite of offices on the third floor in the Roger Main Building became the home of Systems and Procedures on that campus.

Mayo Clinic Jacksonville and St. Luke's Hospital shared the new Systems and Procedures department, with staff and offices being maintained on both campuses.The first staff members to the new section were Mr. Antony Chihak and Ms. Rachel Martin. In 1993 Mr. James Houck joined the team, and an analyst was recruited from State University of New York (SUNY). A number of administrative trainees with post-graduate degrees have rotated through the unit over the years, while gaining valuable experience applied to clinic systems and operations.

Systems and Procedures has served as the in-house consultants for the manual systems and operational processes for the coordination of the many activities involving physicians, patients, and medical information and records, such that the essentials of medical practice are brought together in an appropriate place at a designated time. Founded in 1947, the section worked with the Coordinating Committee on the desk and medical record systems.

Typical projects involved workflow, patient flow, medical record and related information systems, work capacity, and work simplification. Additionally the section has served as a training ground for staff with backgrounds in industrial engineering, administration, finance, and operations research. More recently a new responsibility for continuous improvement, LEAN processes, and analytics is supported from this group.

Dr. Leo F. Black, chief executive officer and chair of the Board of Governors came to me within a few days of my arrival and asked if I could come up with a way to track the clinical capacity to be compared with patient visit volumes. He wanted it organized for the major divisions of Internal Medicine, Surgery, and the Medical Subspecialties. The report I designed for him used the denominator based upon working days in the month. At full capacity, the number of days worked, in the numerator, and working days in the month, in the denominator should match, yielding 100 percent availability. If the physician took time off for vacation, trips, or illness, then availability would be a lower percentage. It provided a means to understand why patient volumes might be off for any given month, and it correlated perfectly with total patient visits and revenue. Once he saw the report and results, he was enthusiastically in support of the new report.

As a former marine, Dr. Black was a forceful figure. The demonstration of the executive information system back at Florida Hospital had a more far-reaching impact that became increasingly clear to me. That experience had given him confidence that he could use an IBM personal computer successfully. As a physician, he had never acquired keyboard skills, so he was a "hunt and peck" typist. He would spend hours (sometimes thirty hours or more over a weekend) building spreadsheets and analyzing the monthly financial and operational statistics reports. The results of his analysis produced questions for his administrative team when he returned from a weekend looking at trends.

During my first year on the job in Jacksonville, an outside consultant engaged by the Arizona practice produced a major systems report. I remember when Dr. Black dropped it off in my office and asked me to look it over to see if there were recommendations that might be applied in Jacksonville. It was a daunting document with hundreds of pages of analysis and recommendations. I remember that as I reviewed it, I saw very few suggestions for efficiency that could be applied successfully to the Jacksonville practice, largely because of the difference in the physical facilities between Florida and Arizona.

There were other problems I found when I started looking, spending time observing various aspects of the operations. One of the more glaring issues I observed is related to the physical structures. Prior to the hospital moving from the original location on the north bank of Jacksonville, near the University of Florida Shands Hospital, a new St. Luke's Hospital was built on Belfort Road on the Southside, with a Friesen design.

Gordon Friesen was an industrial engineer and efficiency expert who worked with a patient care floor plan that called for a nursing unit design based on management engineering principles. Each floor of the hospital had sixty to eighty bed floors, with twenty private rooms on each of the four wings. To get materials from the Central Supply on the ground floor to the floor for patient care, the item would be sent to the Administrative Control Centers (ACC) on each floor via a six-inch pneumatic tube. The ACC was located at the center of the hospital on each patient care floor.

The patient rooms were arranged along both sides of a corridor, with a Team Conference Center (TCC) located midway between the ACC and the end of the hall. At the Administrative Control Center, the shipments were broken down to individual items for each patient. Individual items were then sent via three-inch tubes to the TCCs, about halfway down the corridor for each wing. A TCC was similar to the desk for a nursing unit in a conventional hospital with a conference room, linens, supplies, and a galley.

By the time St. Luke's opened on the Southside around 1980, there were enough changes in leadership that the commitment to the Friesen design was forgotten, the Hospital quickly reverted to the former style of conventional management, and a number of inefficiencies emerged as a result. Mayo Foundation for Medical Education and Research acquired St. Luke's Hospital in 1987, nearly a full year after Mayo Clinic Jacksonville opened.

A typical turn of events of operating in the new facility with the old style of management would take place as follows: A nurse would order an item for a patient. Central Supply would charge the item and send it up to the floor in the six-inch tube where it would arrive in the ACC. Since the cost of staffing the ACC was not sustainable, the room sat empty. The tube would arrive and sit in the inbox. If the ordering nurse was not waiting for it, a nurse from another unit might find the tube, think it was what she ordered, and take it to her patient.

As a result, her patient would not be charged for the item, and the ordering nurse would get to the ACC and find the tube open and the item she ordered gone. She would then call Central Supply to see where the item was. They would report that they had charged the patient and sent it up earlier. There was no option but to reorder the item, and the cycle would begin again.

This is only one example of a number of issues with this design that surfaced once the new hospital was in operation, creating a number of costly inefficiencies. Systems and Procedures studied the system and made recommendations, which resulted in major revisions to the pneumatic tube system to help resolve them. The detailed study traced the thousands of trips to the many nursing stations on all the floors by hours of the day and days of the week to determine the traffic statistics and to estimate the billing errors, lost revenue, and FTE opportunity by improving the system.

In the first few months of operation, we observed that the unit secretary would sit in front of a computer terminal and almost constantly look up lab values for every patient on the unit. When asked about this task, I was told that they had to check for new lab results. When they found a new result, they would transcribe and post it on the patient's chart. When a member of the patient care team checked the chart, they would see the new lab values and notify the physician of the new results.

There was also the associated risk that a numeric value might be transposed, introducing erroneous information and an additional risk to patient care. If it were a critical value, the physician would be called. The computer was fully capable of producing results; however, printers for lab values were not installed on any of the patient care units.

Systems and Procedures produced the plan and cost justification to implement lab printers on each of the nursing units at St. Luke's Hospital. By providing a printer at each of the nursing units, information flow improved for the patient care teams and physicians, and the unit secretary's productivity increased.

In the outpatient setting it was quickly apparent that the growth of the allied health staffing was not sustainable. Every time a new physician joined the staff, a request for a medical secretary and a desk attendant was approved, driving up the overhead for the operation. Systems and Procedures was asked to conduct a major study regarding secretarial work coverage to break this cycle. The completed audit resulted in a major redesign of secretarial job functions and work associated with the support systems.

These examples are a few of the first projects for the new, shared service of Systems and Procedures in Jacksonville. The fundamental challenge went back several years, when Mayo Foundation was deliberating about opening new practices outside of Minnesota. One group felt it was fundamental to the survival of the practice. Dr. Leo F. Black was on the board of governors when the decision was made to open the practice in Florida.

As the section head, I was always concerned that the projects involving a capital request would produce savings, with a projected return on investment within a three- to five-year window. Our team projects made significant improvements and would produce a return on the capital invested; however, with approximately 80 percent of the cost of health care based on payroll, the challenge was clear.

We needed to produce efficiencies that would increase productivity, while reducing the number of allied health staff needed to produce the services. By working together as an administrative team, could we find a way to improve the organization's efficiency and financial performance? Another concern was that Mayo Clinic Jacksonville was adding physician staff at an average rate of approximately fifteen physicians per year. Growing patient panels for that many new physicians in a year is not a trivial task. The leadership team was anxious to increase staff to address the needs for a large integrated group practice. The challenge was to manage both growing the practice and increasing productivity simultaneously. Was that possible?

CHAPTER THREE

Was Continuous Improvement the Answer?

Improve quality, you automatically improve productivity.

—W. Edwards Deming

During that first year, there was a national movement towards quality. It seemed to pervade all industries as a major business focus and priority, stimulated to a large degree by the Malcolm Baldrige National Quality Award, established by the public act of 1987. Awarded by the president, and named in honor of the United States secretary of commerce during the Reagan administration, it is intended to reflect the evolution of the field of quality to focus on overall organizational quality, called performance excellence.

This focus on performance excellence was consistent with the core Mayo Clinic values, and Mr. Carleton Rider, chief administrative officer for the practice, suggested that Mr. Harold Huber, associate administrator, and I attend a weeklong quality improvement seminar in Miami with Dr. Edwards Deming. It was 1992 and Dr. Deming was involved with the post-World War II recovery of Japan, transforming the products manufactured from being cheap and of poor quality to leading products through the continuous quality improvement process. The course materials included his book *Out of the Crisis,* a three-ring binder of syllabus materials, and participant exercises to illustrate the principles used for successful, long-term continuous quality improvement.

The conference days were long, but the content he covered was full of practical information and observations that we felt held huge potential for improving the operations at the Clinic. We returned to work enthusiastic about what we had learned and anxious to apply the process to some operational areas of Mayo Clinic Jacksonville.

Dr. Black was skeptical about the efforts in continuous improvement. Nevertheless, he tolerated our work with the continuous quality improvement (CQI) process in addressing clinical operations.

Systems and Procedures initiated the first continuous improvement project, applying the teamwork methods presented by Dr. Deming. We put together an educational program for the staff, involving the physicians, medical secretaries, desk staff, and operational administration. The Red Bead experiment was used to illustrate the sampling statistical process, and we used a film produced by Joel Barker, futurist and son of a Mayo Clinic staff physician in Rochester, to explain The Business of Paradigms in the introductory program. In the training, we taught the analytical techniques; run charts; the plan, do, check, and analyze (PDCA) steps; root cause analysis; and statistical process controls to bring about change and improvement in the desk system.

The results of that first pilot project in continuous improvement were an overwhelming success. The supervisor of the desk staff for the eighth floor reduced the required staffing level by three full-time equivalents (FTEs) through work simplification and attrition. A number of other changes resulted in improved performances that were tangible to both physicians and patients.

The employees involved in the project were enthusiastic about the process and about being empowered to bring about gradual change and improved efficiency. In the fall of 1992, members of the project team came in to work on a Saturday morning to present and talk about that first pilot project via a two-way video conference with a number of the Clinic leaders in Rochester. The excitement generated was genuine and added credibility to similar processes in Rochester.

The leaders of that first project were invited to present the results to the Board of Governors. A physician leader, the desk supervisor, other key players, and S&P presented an overview of the project, noting the accomplishments of the CQI process and teamwork. We requested permission from the Board to expand the program to other areas of the Clinic.

The third floor physicians and desk staff was next. The acceptance by the staff was positive. Some members were skeptical, but after sitting on the sidelines observing, they soon saw and appreciated the improvements achieved through the CQI, and they joined in with the teams as opportunities arose.

About the time the first successful quality project was completed on the eighth floor desk system, a multi-site Quality Committee was appointed and meetings were instituted on a recurring basis with multi-point video conferencing across the Mayo Clinic sites. Additionally, each site established a physician-led committee to oversee and guide the efforts. The physician director of the Medical Laboratory was appointed to serve on the Foundation-wide committee. A radiologist served as the physician lead for the Quality program in Jacksonville.

As the section head for Systems and Procedures for both the Mayo Clinic and the St. Luke's Hospital, my focus was always on increasing productivity and efficiency in the operations of both sites. Health care systems are comprised of large sets of resources, including human, facility, and equipment. When looking to reduce the cost of operations, facilities and equipment are fixed once the capital has been expended to acquire them. The human resources are very expensive as well but can be somewhat variable through control of staffing (hours worked) and attrition. The CQI program produced results that improved operations and gradually reduced staffing, but it became increasingly clear that the efficiencies needed for Mayo Clinic Jacksonville would require more.

In talking with Dr. Black shortly after starting the job, I mentioned the labor-intensive nature of the paper-based medical record system. In one of our administrative team meetings, I suggested that if the medical record system could be automated, the associated labor savings that would accrue might be significant.

One of the roles of Systems and Procedures is to work with all of the manual processes and make recommendations regarding automation when appropriate. What might seem inappropriate to the reader is that I was not responsible for the information systems serving the practice, so I was in the awkward position of recommending additional work for a colleague's division. I participated as a member of the Information Systems Committee, but a gastroenterologist chaired it at the time, and there was another administrative leader for Information Systems.

Then, unexpectedly, in their meeting on February 12, 1992, the Mayo Clinic Jacksonville Board of Governors established a task force with the following charge: "Recommend to the Board of Governors long-term directions for computerization at Mayo Clinic Jacksonville and review the present availability of applications that might improve clinical practice efficiency at Mayo Clinic Jacksonville."

The group was asked to restrict their deliberations to a philosophical approach and overview of current state-of-the-art information systems. The intention of the directive was to scan the horizon, anticipate future developments, and provide an educational report for the Board by September 1, 1992.

The committee met over the course of six months to evaluate existing systems, meet with vendors, view software demonstrations, and finally, present to the Board of Governors.

The task force was comprised of physicians reflecting a good representation of the specialties in the practice at the time. The information systems administrator and I were the only administrators on the task force. We scheduled meetings at least weekly to discuss and draft what might be in the final report. We were also encouraged by Dr. Black to look at any computer systems or vendors necessary to explore our options for inclusion in our report and recommendations to the Board of Governors. The notion I had discussed with Dr. Black resurfaced, and we began characterizing our goal as attempting the paperless practice of medicine for the outpatient practice.

Once word got out about what we had been asked to do, our colleagues in Rochester decided it was time to update the Information Systems Master Plan, and in July 1992 they convened a Foundation-wide Electronic Medical Record (EMR) Planning Task Force to examine the same issues for the entire practice. A physician from endocrinology was the chair and chairman of the Board of Directors for the Computer-Based Patient Record Institute, Inc. He had also served on the Institute of Medicine, which had developed and written a book about the need for a computer-based patient record (CPR).

An endocrinologist and I represented Mayo Clinic Jacksonville at the meetings by video conference. So now, in addition to the work in Systems and Procedures at two sites, we had two task forces looking at computer automation for the practices. My schedule entailed not only my work and meetings but also travel to visit sites with vendors, looking at products for system automation, and regular video conferences to discuss what was going on at the enterprise level.

There is a fine line between putting in an electronic medical record and attempting the paperless practice of medicine. I used to make this distinction when we later hosted site visits because the question is vitally important.

To the listener I would pose the following question: "If you are not automating to go paperless, then why are you automating?"

The person would often seem stunned by this question. I would continue, "If you are not automating to go paperless, then you are just going to increase the cost of health care. And now you have to maintain dual record systems. That duplicity gets very expensive very quickly and can be the basis for awkward legal situations. Which is your system of record? Is it the computer record or the paper?" Those questions put into perspective what the goal of automation should be.

Fortunately the team assembled in Systems and Procedures was well qualified and able to assist the managers and supervisors with the CQI initiatives. We found a local source for education of the supervisors and required they take an off-site course as a prerequisite for CQI in their work units. Systems and Procedures became a consulting resource to assist with applying the various tools and techniques for supporting the leaders in their various goals and projects. The eighth floor desk staff, and now the third floor, were engaged and using the CQI process to achieve performance improvements and efficiencies.

One of the members of the local automation task force was a member of the St. Luke's Hospital staff before Mayo Foundation acquired it in 1987. He worked with the Cerner Corporation PathNet® Laboratory System and was involved in the original contract negotiations. The Clinic laboratory used a separate competing product at the time. Having been newly appointed to the Mayo Clinic staff, he was facing the technical and logistical challenges of getting both St. Luke's Hospital and Mayo Clinic Jacksonville on a single laboratory information system, and he clearly felt that the Cerner system was superior. His involvement immediately put Cerner on the list of products to be evaluated. With all of these challenges, how would we prioritize? What would happen to the CQI initiatives? How could we sort out the strategy for Mayo Clinic Jacksonville and still try to take the enterprise view for Mayo Foundation?

CHAPTER FOUR

Electronic Medical Record or What?

Experience by itself teaches nothing... Without theory, experience has no meaning. Without theory, one has no questions to ask. Hence, without theory, there is no learning.

—W. Edwards Deming

One of the members of the local task force had experience with the Veterans Administration electronic medical record system and brought a wealth of knowledge about issues that had surfaced in their automated healthcare systems. Perhaps the most notable issue was physician acceptance of using a computer versus the paper-based record, and he warned us repeatedly about usability and acceptance by the clinical staff. The task force took note of his dire warnings and made that a fundamental criterion in our consideration as we evaluated technology solutions.

The next step for our task force was to make an assessment regarding the availability of existing technology. We invited the principals from Cerner Corporation to visit Mayo Clinic Jacksonville and meet with the task force to share information. CEO Neal Patterson and the chief medical officer for Cerner made the trip and spent time touring both Mayo Clinic and St. Luke's Hospital.

The chief medical officer outlined the various information services in use at the time. The traditional model was prevalent from the early '70s and was characterized with the financial system as core with the registration, order entry, and accounts receivable. Other systems typically connected by batched or interfaced entry might include laboratory, radiology, pharmacy, materials management (logistics), dietary, respiratory, quality assurance/utilization review, and others. That was the prevalent model of information architecture for many health care systems of the time.

The establishment of the network model of information architecture for computer workstations began to grow in the early 1980s, and my prior experience included the establishment of the first networking of personal computer workstations at Florida Hospital in 1981. And within a decade, networking grew exponentially. With the advent of networking technology, the notion of tying applications together via networks became in vogue. Mayo was a participant in this movement as one of the founders of the Health Level 7 (HL7), with membership in the HL7 standards development group.

The HL7 group was created with the intent of developing an industry-wide standard for making applications interact without the need to develop custom interfaces for each application. Problems with this interface tended to stem from different vendors interpreting the standards as they perceived them. Once the applications were installed, additional programming effort was sometimes required to "clean up" the HL7 interface for the new applications. The underlying assumption for this architecture was that as clinical needs are identified, the network can be expanded to include new applications at a minimum of expense and difficulty.

The third information architecture was characterized as the loosely coupled data repository, which was driven in part by the advent of relational database technology in the early '80s. The popularity of relational database technology or structured query language (SQL) for the development of new applications was driven by the relative ease of creation, maintenance, and expansion of data structure. This development spawned the loosely coupled data repository as the foundation around which many applications can be built.

Rochester Information Services pursued that architecture at the time, with the Electronic Results Inquiry System (ERIS) as the first venture in the design. As implied by its name, the loosely coupled architecture is relative to the other models and derives its name from systems that are fairly independent while producing their final results into a common data repository that can be accessed by other systems.

The degree of integration achieved by this model is superior to that offered by the earlier two models, but it was not as advanced as the fourth and final model in the discussion of systems architectures.

The final model was the tightly coupled systems architecture, also known as fully integrated. The benefits of the tightly coupled architecture were derived from the ability to actively interchange information between the various component systems in a uniform common user interface. The integrated architecture was an ideal, and to the best information available to the task force, there was no one software vendor that could deliver this architectural model in a complete form at the time, so it represented a goal of information systems designers, rather than a reality. The chief medical officer, as a spokesperson for the Cerner Corporation, willingly acknowledged that his company could not deliver this system, although they believed they were substantially on their way to building this comprehensive application suite.

Since then, the client-server information architecture has arrived, and the Internet now reflects the emergence and maturity of the networked models of today. Just as building architecture evolved, these four models represented different views towards information systems. But building architecture has existed for centuries, whereas automated healthcare information systems have only been in existence for approximately thirty years.

Briefly identifying the various Mayo entities and their relative positions in these architectural timelines, Mayo Clinic Jacksonville and Scottsdale were clearly the traditional information architectures at the time since they were largely financially driven with lab reporting being an ancillary system.

With the advent of Electronic Results Inquiry System (ERIS), which was based upon the architecture of the PHAMIS Last Word architecture, they took a step forward toward the loosley coupled information systems architecture.

During our discussions with the Cerner leadership, they asked what we were trying to accomplish through automation. Dr. Black made it abundantly clear that we were interested in automation as a means of saving money! We were not pursuing it because we wanted to prove anything or beat anyone else to the punch. The need to save money was driven by his perceived need to get the Florida practice financially improved.

The folks from Cerner were amazed and said they had never met with any group or organization that wanted to automate to save money. That was simply unheard of in the health care computer industry as a stated objective. They welcomed the opportunity to work to accomplish our objectives.

As a task force, we had just scratched the surface of our search for a potential technology partner. We needed to draft a vision to serve as a reference point for evaluating vendors and products. After many meetings and much discussion, we settled on the following needs and requirements for our automation efforts.

The goal of increased efficiency for Mayo Clinic Jacksonville could be most effectively met through automation of the most labor-intensive tasks that created the most delays.

The Medical Record. The unit record in use at Mayo Clinic was designed to document and communicate the findings. As the repository for all of a patient's clinical information, it was the *primary point of contention* for those who needed access to it.

Automation of the medical record needed to produce efficiencies through providing a means for simultaneous access by multiple persons, adding to the record through various means, and reducing the number of paramedical staff involved in processing the medical record.

Movement between the Clinic and Hospital. Since St. Luke's Hospital was ten miles from Mayo Clinic, travel time had a dramatic impact on productivity, which at the time was greater than that of the other two Mayo entities. The ability of a physician to check on an inpatient's progress via an electronic terminal would have a profound impact on productivity.

Physician Work Flow. Automation of communication to the medical record would enhance physician efficiency and improve patient satisfaction through the following features.

- **Phyician Input of Orders and Charges**. Studies of the turnaround time for Scheduling Services documented in the Continuous Improvement Patient Encounter Task Force revealed more than an hour's delay in returning an itinerary to the patient once the MSR was available and sent to Scheduling Services.
- **Speech Recognition.** Efforts to use voice recognition technology for physician notes would eliminate the need for transcription pools for adding notes to history. The institution needed to continue to develop rapid turnaround dictation/transcription systems in order to capture textual information in ways that it could be inserted directly into an electronic record.
- **X-ray Tracking**. X-ray tracking had been in operation at Jacksonville since mid-December 1991 and had proven very effective in reducing the amount of delay produced by misdirected or lost X-rays.
- **Resources**. Resource utilization analysis would permit physicians within specialty or sub-specialty groups to compare clinical performance for similar diagnoses.

Performance Data Collection. As systems should become progressively automated, and key processes should collect data automatically to support the collection needs of the Continuous Improvement Process teams.

Referring Physicians. As Mayo Clinic Jacksonville grew, it would become increasingly important to build referring physician linkages with outside primary care specialists. Sharing diagnostic materials with the patient's primary physician would make him or her a partner with Mayo Clinic.

Prioritizing Advanced Appointments. The central appointment process could be more effective with system assistance in recognizing patients who will most benefit from Mayo Clinic care and the degree of urgency for appointments.

Scheduling of Tests, Procedures, and Consults. Rules-based scheduling of consults, tests, and procedures must be required to assure appropriate sequencing and optimum timing of patient appointments.

Generation of Correspondence. Future systems must reduce effort of physicians and secretaries when producing letters following episodes of care.

With the statement of these goals, the groundwork for our challenge became clearer. Where would they take us? Could we put an information architecture in place that would enable Mayo Clinic Jacksonville to reduce its resource requirements to the point that the operational return would improve? Did these goals suggest something bigger than an electronic medical record? Could Cerner, or any other information systems company, put such a system in place?

CHAPTER FIVE

Imaging Systems and Evaluations

If you can't describe what you are doing as a process, you don't know what you're doing.

—W. Edwards Deming

In June of 1992, I traveled to San Diego to the Association of Information and Image Management (AIIM) annual conference and exposition. In a most rudimentary form, a good imaging system should be capable of making a full copy of a paper-based medical record, indexing it, and delivering it wherever needed for patient care. New information could be handwritten or transcribed, imaged, and added to the repository and circulated to the patient care team. Today's flat LED screens did not exist back then. A standard imaging system recommended a twenty-one- or twenty-two-inch, high-resolution monitor in order to make the image comfortably readable for the user. The scanner resolution needed to be two hundred dots per inch, because storage space for the resulting image would use up relatively expensive storage media.

When I returned from that trip, I had seen enough of the technology and the attendant workflow automation to be convinced there was a way to take the practice of medicine paperless, even if it needed to be done with a good imaging system. Later that month and quite by surprise, I was informed that the Board of Governors had made me the Chair of the Division of Systems Support Services. My new division consisted of Systems and Procedures, Information Services, and Telecommunications for the Mayo Clinic Jacksonville operation. The new role put me in an awkward position of chairing Information Services at the Clinic but not at St. Luke's Hospital, because at that time I had the responsibility for the Clinic campus but not the Hospital. The director of Information Services at the Hospital would report to me at the Clinic but not at the Hospital.

As the task force was evaluating technology, IBM offered to bring in one of their imaging systems to try an experiment. We decided to have them convert seventy-five medical records by the scanning and indexing process, and then make them available online. They set up a terminal for the imaging system in one of the meeting rooms off the main dining room in the cafeteria. Dr. Black brought in physician thought leaders, one at a time, let them review a chart, and asked them a number of questions regarding the quality of the image for readability and about the suitability of the system in regards to practicing medicine. He asked them if it worked well enough to no longer send them the paper-based record.

The results were nearly unanimous in the affirmative, that it was possible. How to input the records was not well thought out; however, there was agreement that it would work, assuming a good method for entering records could be contrived. I think that from that point on, he was convinced that my proposal to take the practice paperless was feasible, but we needed more data about the projected savings.

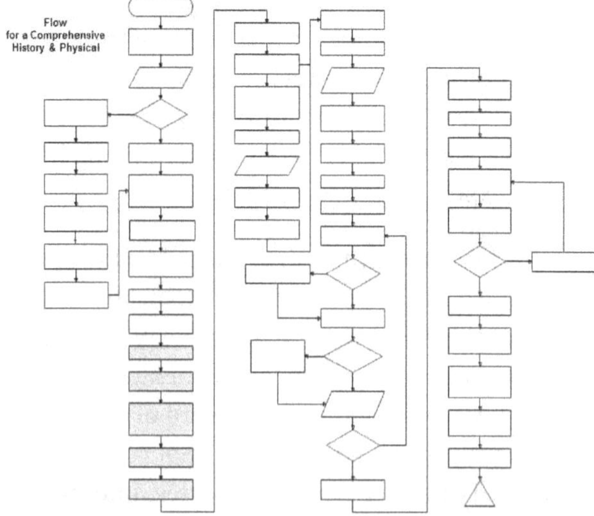

Used with permission of Mayo Foundation for Medical Education and Research, all rights reserved.

Mr. Tony Chihak in Systems and Procedures prepared detailed workflow analyses of the three most universal appointment types at the time: the comprehensive history and physical (CHP), the specialty consults (SPEC), and the return visit (RTNV). The detail of the workflow would yield the number of steps in the manual processing of the paper-based medical record. Then, based upon the plan for going paperless, we prepared detailed workflow analyses for the remaining work after the automation was complete. With these comparisons, we could work with the supervisor of each desk area to assess the number of staff that would be required if we eliminated the work associated with the paper-based medical record system.

The above diagram details the steps in the process for the paper-based medical record system at the time, beginning with the patient calling in for an appointment with a physician for a comprehensive history and physical exam. The blocks highlighted in gray reflect the time the patient spent with the physician, which is the only part of the process for which revenue is collected. The other steps in the process reflect activities for allied health staff (part of the Clinic overhead costs), and it is relatively fixed with the staffing model.

The following diagram reflects the same diagram, but the items marked with black diagonal stripes on the gray background reflect potential work that could be eliminated with the paperless practice of medicine. As a crude measure, it would eliminate approximately

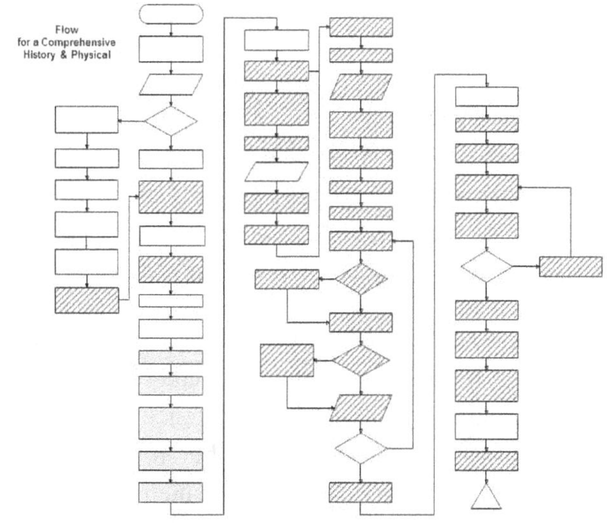

50 percent of the associated labor.

Similar diagrams were prepared for the specialty consults, appointments where an appropriate specialist sees and evaluates a patient for a particular problem. For example, the physician performing the CHP might refer a patient who complains of chest pains for further evaluation by a cardiologist.

The final step in the Mayo Clinic process results in a return visit with the physician who performed the CHP. By the time this visit happens, all of the clinical findings and evaluations are routed back to the CHP physician, who then spends time with the patient reviewing the findings, providing proper context, and developing a plan with the patient based upon recommendations from the clinical findings. In some cases, an urgent or emergent need may be discovered and corrective surgery scheduled for the next day, or as soon as possible.

Our projected benefits based upon our workflow analysis for all three appointment types were: The CHP manual processing would be reduced from fifty-five to twenty-five steps, SPEC manual processing reduced from forty to seventeen steps, and RTNV manual processing reduced from twenty-nine to nineteen steps. On one hand, not every patient went through all three of these processes once. The specialty consults often happened in accordance with the number of problems that might have surfaced in the CHP or other SPEC appointments. Our generalization was that the eliminated work would amount to half or more of those areas involved in the paper-based medical record handling, so the impact would fall on Medical Records, the desk staff, Report Summary and Completion, and medical secretaries. These groups reflected a sizeable amount of the allied health staff, and the potential savings (wages and benefits) might be significant.

The value of the work of Mr. Tony Chihak in documenting these process flows and steps cannot be underestimated. His work was brilliant and clearly explained the difference in the automation and manual processes. Comparing the before-and-after steps, in addition to the parts of the process where medicine is practiced and revenue generated, crystallized the changes being sought. Our team was fortunate to have Tony as a member, and he brought freshness to Systems and Procedures, having been hired as a new graduate from the University of Wisconsin at the same time I joined Mayo Clinic.

With these projections, the next steps in our analysis would be to examine the volumes for each appointment type, number of full-time equivalents for each area, human resources, and benefits, all on an annual basis to establish the potential impact on the operational expenses.

The administration continued to fight the budgetary crunch. While we were making the case for the automation of the clinical practice, the St. Luke's Hospital administrative staff asked Systems and Procedures if we could identify efficiencies within hospital operations that would make a significant contribution to the bottom line. Would it be better to engage an outside consultant for the assessment? If we agreed to do the assessment; however, it would forever change the perception of Systems and Procedures as an in-house consulting group with the supervisors and managers, thus limiting our effectiveness long term. It would have cast Systems and Procedures in the role of "head hunters;" if we looked at an operational issue in a section or department, employees would have feared that their jobs would be eliminated.

An outside consulting group was engaged to conduct what was called Operational Excellence, or OE. Dr. Black led the teams and supported the effort. Still, we knew from our discussions with Dr. Black that he held a degree of skepticism about the project, but he wanted it to work. If it worked for the Hospital, we knew he would consider it for the Clinic. At this point, automation as a means to reduce expenses had potential, but automation to save money was still an unknown and unproven means of reducing expenses in health care. Historically it had driven up the cost of health care due to the large capital expenses and ongoing maintenance fees. The consulting team of analysts examined every aspect of hospital operations, and they made recommendations for changes that would produce improvement in the Hospital's bottom line.

Objectives and financial targets were set. Members of the leadership team were assigned to groups, and numerous meetings were convened to brainstorm ideas that could be implemented to reduce expenses or increase income, with the goal of ultimately improving St. Luke's Hospital's bottom line. Over the ensuing year, goals were met, finances improved, and staff reductions were made through natural attrition. While the Hospital was engaged in Operations Efficiency, the Clinic staff of Systems and Procedures worked to build better projections for the improvement that could be produced by automation at the Clinic.

Automation of systems is complex work that requires time, especially if it involves a change in the culture of the organization. Expecting a physician to key in his or her clinical notes via computer was not realistic. Most physicians at the time had no training in the use of a keyboard. The legibility of handwritten notes by physicians was a problem of the paper-based system. We had to find a way to make it more efficient for our physicians to input the clinical notes.

Physicians already used dictation for Radiology, Surgery, Anesthesia, and several other subspecialties. Since the technology was already in use, we began to consider how to make it a utility, available for all physicians regardless of their specialty.

Ordering for patients was well organized with an eight-page booklet called the Medical Service Record (MSR). Systems and Procedures worked with the Coordinating Committee on revision and publication of the booklet every six months. The paper-based ordering system of all procedures, diagnostic tests, evaluations, and consults which could be ordered for a patient. There was one, sometimes more, MSR used for each patient, and it became a part of the packet contained in the medical record while the chart was active. An integral part of the automation would need to address this aspect of the workflow.

Obviously there would be a significant impact on medical records, since over time more and more of the clinical data would be collected from automated systems and never produced on paper. We postulated that, ideally, all clinical information needed to be stored in a discrete database for the greatest utility of the numeric values that would be contained there.

As systems staff, we took a fundamental approach to what the electronic medical record might resemble as we tried to capitalize on existing systems, adding components that would be robust and scalable to support the paperless practice of medicine. The existing systems we wanted to leverage included CyCare (the fundamental business system), used to open the practice at Mayo Clinic Jacksonville. The clinical laboratory system in use was Sunquest.

In talking with Carl Rider, chief administrative officer at the time, about why the information systems in Rochester were not used in the opening of the practice, I learned that he had asked for their systems and support, but they didn't have the infrastructure capacity at the time. Carl had worked on the opening of the new practice in Jacksonville as a member of Systems and Procedures in Rochester, prior to being relocated and appointed administrator. He always had a positive outlook and a can-do attitude that I found reassuring in going about my work.

The task force concluded that the paperless effort we envisioned would need additional systems for transcription and dictation for the addition of new clinical information and an imaging system to provide support of images of the paper medical record. We felt it imperative to visit and study sites already attempting the transition from paper-based to electronic medical records.

The challenge was how to leverage existing automated systems with additional supporting systems to complete the automation. Was it even possible?

CHAPTER SIX

Medical Record Logistics

With tens of thousands of patients dying every year from preventable medical errors, it is imperative that we embrace available technologies and drastically improve the way medical records are handled and processed.

—Jon Porter, Congressman

My predecessors started the quest for efficiency in the practice with one notable effort, operating as the Medical Records Task Force. In the paper-based medical record environment, the pivotal piece of information is the location of the record and who is in charge of it. In attempts to keep it moving, there was a whole series of rules regarding the circulation of the medical record.

For example, the four-hour rule stated that a patient appointment requiring the medical record could not be scheduled without an interval of four hours. If a patient was being seen at 10 a.m., the earliest he could be seen that same day would be at 2 p.m. This interval would allow time for the physician to handwrite his or her findings in the medical record and have it routed on to the location for the following appointment. The interval was two hours if the appointment did not require the medical record to be available for reference.

There was a twenty-four-hour rule for appointments between the Clinic and Hospital. So if a patient was seen at the Clinic, and then needed to be at the Hospital for her next diagnostic procedure or exam, it had to be scheduled for the next day. It didn't matter that a patient might be able to get in his car and shortly be ten miles down the road, parked, and ready to be seen in one hour. The logistics of getting the medical record ready for the following appointment might require the added work of a handwritten or transcribed note, and then someone would have to transport it to the other site. General services rotated vans back and forth with lab specimens, medical records, and X-rays between sites almost continuously. One exception was in the case of a patient booked for next-day surgery.

Special handling of the medical record was involved for next-day surgery. The same was not true for patients who were discharged and needed to be seen in the outpatient setting at the Clinic. Their appointments would be scheduled for the next day at the earliest. There was a very complex set of rules with regard to the medical record due to the time delay created by physicians and clinicians needing to add information to the paper-based medical record and then get it moved to the next point of care.

One of the challenges was the task of putting the medical record sheets in the proper order. The Plummer record had evolved to a complex set of documents created by Systems and Procedures, working with the Coordinating Committee, over the years. The reason behind all of the specialized forms was physician efficiency, with the focus of the forms often based on a specialty or special needs for clinical information. The outer wrap of the record was the master sheet, which included the current registration information for the patient. Lab results were attached to the lab folio with shingle sheets, and radiology results were similarly arranged.

Other specialty sheets included such items as electrocardiograms, urology, cardiology, otorhinolaryngology, to name a few of the nearly three hundred fifty medical record forms we stopped printing eventually. The medical record fit into a plastic jacket with pockets on the outside that contained the routing information. The size of the forms were approximately 6.25 by 9 inches for a half sheet, 12.5 by 9 inches for a full sheet, and the master sheet was the equivalent of three half sheets (18.75 by 9 inches), folded in thirds. With the standard for paper now 8.5 by 11 inches, finding printers to fit the original forms would have been prohibitively expensive.

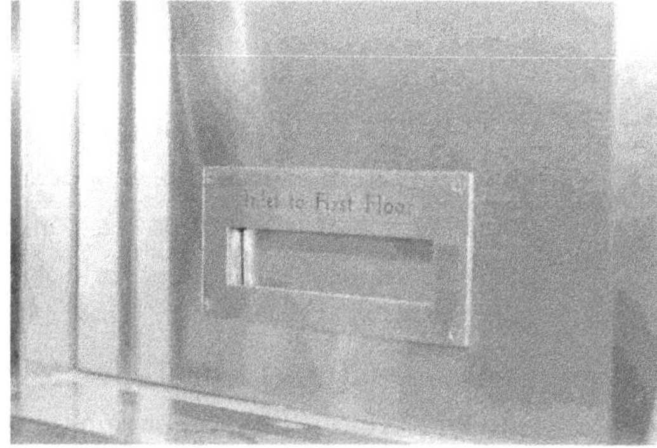

Medical record input to the chute system.

Historically the vertical building architecture used gravity to assist in the circulation of the paper-based medical record. In Jacksonville there was a lift system to convey the medical records and X-rays up to the floor where the patient was being seen.

When the medical record needed to be moved to a new location, a desk attendant would put a new routing slip in the pocket on the plastic packet and then drop it down a chute to Medical Records on the ground floor of the Davis Building. When the chutes were installed in the Davis Building, the medical records came out of the chute so fast that they skidded across the floor. A bin was added at the end of the chute to catch the medical record as they came out of the chute. Still too fast, a mechanical brake was added in the final curve of the chute to slow the descent of the medical record packet.

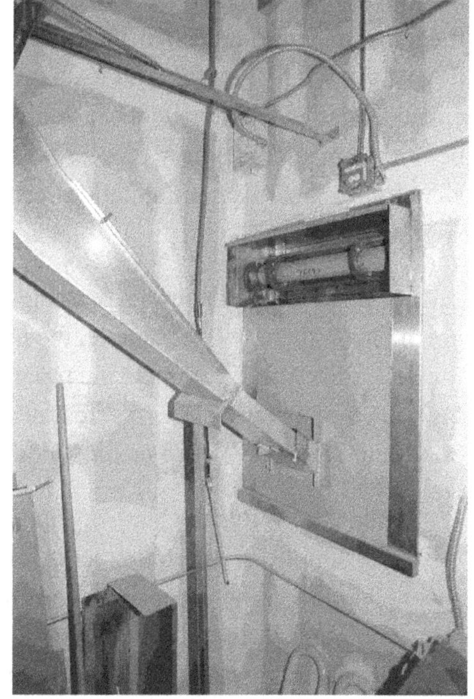

Behind the scene look at the end of the chute in Medical Records.

The Medical Records Task Force worked on a number of issues. The list included:

- Getting the desk staff to put the medical record in the proper order before giving it to the physician,
- Getting clinicians to use both sides of the progress notes to conserve space (an unintended consequence of this tactic was that information might be overlooked by not reading the backside of the notes),
- Consolidating the hospital episode of care (EOC) information into an envelope, and other related issues.

There was a Report and Summary section when I started at Mayo Clinic Jacksonville. The main task was to consolidate information to make the paper forms more efficient for the physicians to use. Staff members would take the individual lab result sheets and transcribe them by hand onto green lab summary sheets. The backlog in this section was typically months, and it was common for a record to be called from the department because the patient had returned to be seen before the record summary process was completed. Radiology results were transcribed from the shingle sheets onto a summary sheet for that specialty.

On desks where there was ongoing care, oncology patients undergoing chemotherapy for example, the history rarely left the floor, and the desk staff would complete the report summary task on site. The logistics of the paper-based medical record distracted from the more important issues involving medical practice.

When Drs. Will and Charlie Mayo started practicing, they used a relatively simple set of requirements for their medical records (journals at the time). The purpose of their medical records was to track the most important facts and findings associated with patient care, with the goal of retrospective review and evaluation to learn about their practice, including the more important discoveries over time.

The basic data set that I observed included the patient name, general address, age, gender, presenting complaint, findings, treatment, and outcome, usually stated in a succinct, handwritten paragraph. There were no insurance companies or third-party payers, Joint Commission, Medicare, or Medicaid. Current medicine requires meeting expectations—if it isn't documented, it wasn't done.

Our litigious attitudes require that physicians practice defensive medicine to rule out anything possibly overlooked. In many cases, the cost of medical care now covers tests that are likely to reveal little additional information, but failure to order the tests might be construed as an error of omission in a court trial.

Recently a physician wrote a letter to *The Wall Street Journal* decrying the waste of resources consumed by forcing physicians to implement electronic medical records in their practices. His specialty is anesthesia, and his medical treatment of patients is critical to their well-being, primarily while they are under anesthesia.

The anesthesia record documents what was done to treat the patient while in his care, but quickly becomes an artifact once the patient has safely recovered. The point is that different practices have a broad spectrum of medical record requirements that are driven by their practice needs. The anesthetist needs an automated medical record capable of real-time charting of multiple data observations intraoperatively. Afterwards, a concise summary will fill the needs for most of the other physicians involved in caring for the patient.

Contrast that with the needs of the general internist conducting a history and physical on a "worried well" patient. Today there are very strict guidelines for documentation of the findings, such as presenting complaint, family history, social history, review of systems, physical findings, recommendations, etc.

Finally, for reimbursement, the documentation must include level of effort (five possible levels), time spent in counseling, and so on. The requirements change frequently, and if the documentation is not up to standard, reimbursement for the visit will be denied. Mayo Clinic, a large integrated group practice, requires the complex medical record logistics that are described here. For the vital pieces of information in the record, it was essential to move it from place to place for the patient. The medical record access policy at the time stated that the medical record was the property of Mayo Clinic and should not be removed from the record keeping system. The patient should not be given an opportunity to read the medical record.

The American Health Insurance Portability and Accountability Act of 1996 (HIPAA) forced Mayo Clinic to change the medical record access policy to meet the requirements of rules to be followed by doctors, hospitals and other health care providers. The law helps ensure that all medical records, medical billing, and patient accounts meet certain consistent standards with regard to documentation, handling, and privacy. Exclusive ownership of the medical record by the health care provider ended, and patients were given the right to their own information. This development in 1996 has greatly benefited patients to allow them to engage in managing their own health.

The needs of the medical record had evolved from the early days of the Mayo Clinic practice to the remarkably complex levels of documentation required today. Given the complexity of the paper-based medical record, could it be automated? Would physicians be disposed to using the computer-based medical record? What would be the impact on their practices if it could be done?

CHAPTER SEVEN

Paperless Requirements

I don't understand, given the constraints physicians have in doing their job and the paperwork demanded of them, why people want to be physicians. I think we've made it very, very difficult for them to perform their job. I think that's a shame.

—Malcolm Gladwell
Forbes, March 13, 2014

It is important to understand that what was proposed was the paperless practice of medicine as opposed to the implementation of an electronic medical record. As our task force in Jacksonville worked on the means to automate the practice, our colleagues in Rochester and Arizona focused on an essential ingredient: the electronic medical record. From a systems perspective, the approach in Jacksonville was broader and more holistic. We treated the process for the work of the physician as comprised of a set of activities that included review of the previous clinical record, ordering, scheduling with instructions, charging, and then the documentation of findings and results in the computer-based medical record.

A patient encounter at Mayo Clinic typically starts with a request for an appointment by a potential patient. There is a common misconception that one must be referred to Mayo Clinic by a physician in order to make an appointment. In fact, 80 percent of the patients are self-referred, which means that they believe they have a problem and would like to be evaluated by a Mayo Clinic consultant. The Central Appointment Office (CAO) takes the call, and then on the basis of symptoms and/or complaints, will set up an appointment with a physician for an evaluation. Previous medical X-rays, consultant findings, or other clinical results may be requested prior to the actual appointment. With few exceptions, the appointment will be the key pivotal event from which the bulk of clinical work and revenue will result. Our attempt at the automation of the clinical practice was focused on trying to get full accountability for the entire practice.

Full accountability was challenging at best due to the amount of administrative paperwork associated with providing the clinical care. By automating and tracking the process with computer technology, we believed the appointment would either be met, cancelled, or re-scheduled. If the patient met the appointment with the scheduled physician, then there would be a corresponding charge for the visit. It was likely that additional diagnostic tests, procedures, and consults would be ordered and subsequently scheduled. The charge for the appointment should flow into the revenue recognition system, with appropriate diagnoses and billing codes, and a clinical note of the findings should be charted in the computer system and available for the downstream processes.

One problem we were trying to improve was lost or misplaced orders and charge sheets. As a part of administration, we believed that the loose-leaf nature of the practice was causing the Clinic to lose some amount of revenue. With a good ordering and scheduling system, the accountability for all of the outpatient practice through automation should be 100 percent, or nearly so. In our systems work, we had discovered that occasionally someone had an accident with, or misplaced, the charge sheets, resulting in lost charges. Similar problems happened with the orders placed with the medical service requisition (MSR) booklets.

In desperation, a clinician might grab another booklet and place more orders. The resulting duplicate order booklet, along with the missing MSR when discovered, generated more questions and confusion about duplicate orders, or which one needed to be used for the actual ordering in the system. Of course duplicate orders for the same test is wasteful, as is missing a test necessary to confirm a diagnosis because of a misplaced booklet.

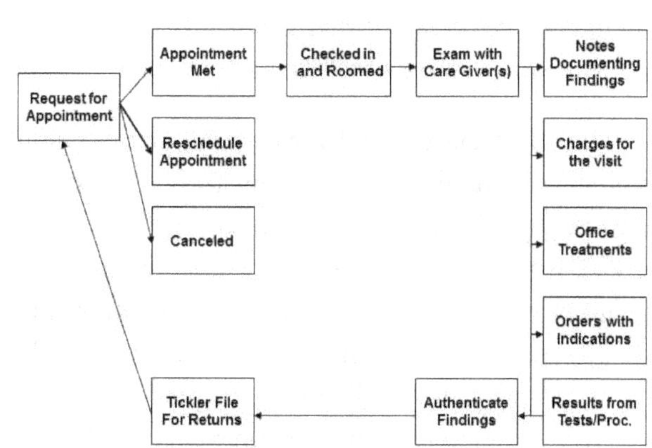

Conceptually it was what we termed *closing the clinical loop*, illustrated by the following diagram. The process starts with the request for an appointment and the subsequent scheduling. The possibility of cancelling or rescheduling is provided. Upon arrival for the appointment, the patient is checked in, roomed as an exam room is available, and then seen by the physician.

Following the exam, the physician creates the clinical notes of the findings, charges, results, orders for additional tests and consults and, in some cases, an office treatment may be provided. The results from all of the tests, consults, and/or procedures are routed back to the ordering physician.

The option for a return visit is not explicitly shown on this diagram, but it is an essential part of providing feedback to the patient regarding the findings, course of treatment, and patient education regarding his health, plus mapping a strategy that would include engaging the patient in activities that might be beneficial in managing his health status. It's this final step in the process of engaging the patient in activities that need to be addressed. The task force was convinced that by closing this loop, full accountability or very near full accountability, could be achieved.

In the course of our deliberation and planning, a number of principles emerged that we found useful in guiding the development and goals for our recommendations. The first principle was that *automa-*

tion to become an integrated healthcare delivery system requires the information systems to be built with an integrated architecture.

The complexity of delivering health care is considerably more challenging than that of other industries. For example, the process of delivering products at organizations such as Amazon or United Parcel Service is relatively straightforward. A given item is picked from an inventory of products, prepared for shipment, routed to a transportation system, which in turn, moves it across a distribution network where it is ultimately delivered to the end consumer. Tools, which operate over telecommunication systems and the Internet, enable tracking the product to its destination. There is little or no transformation on the product once it is picked from inventory, with the exception of the preparation for shipment and the charging mechanism.

Contrast that with the health care system where a patient is seen, evaluated, given additional tests as measures of health, or for diagnostic purposes, may be the subject of a transformative process such as surgery to remove an inflamed appendix or hospitalization. The process is infinitely more complex with more steps, exceptions, treatments, morbidities, or comorbidities. With more interactions automated between information systems, the greater the possibility of efficiencies within the organizations.

An example of the interactions between systems would be to examine each medication prescribed by the physician to check for the possibility of patient sensitivities or allergies, or to check for drug-drug interactions, which may be detrimental to the patient's condition. The use of systems with an integrated architecture greatly helps the organization in achieving improved patient safety and long-term economies. This is fundamental to obtain the maximum efficiencies for the users in meeting the goals of the enterprise.

It is generally well recognized in the United States that physician compensation is in the top tier of income-earning categories; therefore, the cost of those wages make the physician a very expensive resource in any practice setting. The second principle is the fundamental rule of business economics wherein *optimization of the system must be directed toward improving the effectiveness of the most expensive resources,* making the physician the pivotal resource to be addressed.

Our automation efforts were directed towards making the computer system as effective in meeting the physicians' needs as possible. Bringing software engineers into the exam room whenever possible proved to be an excellent way to impress software developers of who the client was as we worked on software engineering. Physicians, as one of the most expensive resources, are the key to gaining the most cost-effective model of care.

At Mayo Clinic, the preeminent corporate value is that the needs of the patient come first, and a hallmark of the practice and key to patient satisfaction is quality time with the physician. The third principle was directed at *automation of the mundane parts of the physician practice*. This principle enables more and better time with the patient. Writing notes and completing documentation are undoubtedly the mundane tasks and regarded as clerical work by many physicians. This is especially true if physicians are expected to write their clinical notes using a keyboard. The task force knew that if we expected manual entry by physicians, the project of automating was doomed at the outset.

Ironically the Plummer paper-based medical records in use at Mayo Clinic at the time required physicians to handwrite their clinical findings on the loose-leaf paper pages or specialty sheets. The industrial engineering adage of "handle it once" was a key ingredient of the success of the paper-based record, which had been in use for eighty-five years. It worked best because the physician was encouraged to write the notes while in the exam room with the patient, or before moving on to see the next patient.

The efficiency of the paper-based record dropped quickly if the physician did not complete his or her notes soon after the patient encounter. We knew that no one aspires to practice medicine for the record keeping duties required of the profession. The goal was to minimize that activity. This aspect was going to be a critical part of the automation of the practice.

The fourth principle guiding our efforts was that *medical information regarding patient tests had a time decay factor*. Automation efforts had to support the timely flow of information to the care provider to enhance patient care. As more integration of the systems occurred, the improved timeliness of results would enhance care. As more and more results become available electronically, the greater the physician acceptance of automation.

In converting a paper-based medical record system, we assumed that all results were analog in nature. Digital results, such as those from the laboratory system, would ideally flow into the computer-based record. Imaging was the means to capture all the rest of the analog forms. Over time, more and more of the information generated on a patient would flow directly into the computer-based system and less would be based on the analog paper images. The timeliness of the information was critical, and it needed to flow quickly, accurately, and unimpeded.

The fifth principle guiding the work of our task force was that *building an integrated healthcare delivery system required a long-term relationship with a technology partner, with both deriving benefits from the relationship*. Building a critical database to serve the needs of the health care provider is not a trivial task, and once established, it would grow into a very large repository.

Health care is a dynamic business, and the needs grow over time, requiring new applications, new database schema, software upgrades, capital outlays, and staffing. We had to view it as a long-term investment, and migration to a new vendor could prove to be a huge obstacle. The task force was convinced that Mayo Clinic Jacksonville needed to build a relationship with a technology partner as a strategic alliance, because it would have profound benefits to both organizations.

The final principle was to *provide a structure to the computer-based medical record that resembled the existing paper-based Plummer record as an exact replica.* The physicians, who had spent years with the Plummer records, knew that following the Master sheet, they would find the Laboratory Summary with the most recent findings first, followed by a summary of the Radiology results, and so on. It would have been much more complex to attempt to restructure the record to something less familiar.

With our paperless requirement goals established and the principles formulated, we faced the next set of problems. What would we do to get our clinical notes into the computer-based electronic medical records we were proposing? Would our physicians adapt to using the computer-based medical record? What would be the impact on physician productivity? Could we accomplish our goals without turning our physicians into highly compensated "clerks"?

Our project was facing a long list of challenges to overcome if we were going to be successful.

CHAPTER EIGHT

Projected Labor Reductions

When we cooperate, everybody wins.

—W. Edwards Deming

The task force quickly became convinced that the automation of the clinical practice would gain a number of efficiencies; however, if we were going to assemble a serious project and get the needed capital, we would have to assemble some projections for the labor reductions that would accrue. My team in Systems and Procedures had built the detailed steps reflecting the current work and the labor requirement, assuming a successful project through automation. We were asked to complete a detailed analysis with each of the areas that would be affected by the automation.

We built a list of all the work units involved with the process for the medical record. The list of staffing included Medical Records, the desk, Report Summary and Completion, General Services, and Patient Accounts. In January of 1992, the approved full-time equivalents in these areas amounted to 187 positions. We met with each of the work unit supervisors to discuss staffing requirements for their area, assuming we were successful in eliminating the circulation of the paper-based medical record.

Everyone agreed that omitting the need to sort and circulate the medical record would result in the elimination of additional work and the associated staff. By the time we concluded our assessment, we projected that more than half of the staff could be eliminated, if we stopped circulating the medical record and moved to the electronic medical record. This included automating the medical record the attendant forms for ordering of tests and consults, and the professional service charge sheets.

Administration discussed how to reduce staffing without resorting to layoffs. These talks led to a plan to replace staff for these areas with limited tenure positions as turnover occurred. From our work in systems, we knew that once work was eliminated, the organization had to be ready to take the savings rather than look for other work the staff could do to fill their time. With the limited tenure positions, there would be no repercussions when the supervisor had to let them go. Those employees knew their jobs were not guaranteed. Despite the limited tenure positions, we had no problem filling them on an interim basis.

The task force made its report to the Board of Governors in September 1992, with no definitive action taken immediately.

The conclusions and recommendations of the task force are summarized here.

- The Mayo Clinic and St. Luke's Hospital should replace current systems with integrated Clinic-Hospital systems with an integrated architecture.
- New systems should be tightly integrated, while allowing some interfacing as well. A model using tightly integrated core applications should be adopted if a suitable vendor partnership could be defined. Core applications included registration/admission-discharge-transfer (ADT), appointments, ordering, scheduling, care planning, and all components of an electronic medical record (EMR).
- Systems that support ancillary departments should use the integrated database wherever possible. The systems architecture should provide easy-to-implement interfacing methods for patient demographics, schedules, charges, results, and other

data. Clinical systems had to contribute findings directly to an EMR.

- The cost-effectiveness of new systems should be managed. It was important to choose a partner who was both able and committed, to meet our needs long-term.
- The conversion would be expensive in terms of human effort—physicians, administration, and all allied health staff—as well as equipment and software development.
- Updating and movement of paper medical records was expensive, and maintaining that cost while at the same time processing an electronic record was redundant. The EMR should incorporate existing paper records to enable full electronic movement.
- Developments should be phased, but the vision must be clear. Implementation of new systems would involve risk, particularly at the early stages. Pilot and demonstration projects should be defined wherever possible.
- Operational systems and the EMR should work in conjunction with one another.
- The Jacksonville plan should be compatible with Mayo Foundation. The information systems plan for Mayo Clinic Jacksonville needed to be an integral part of the long-term Mayo Foundation strategic plan as well. The Foundation should take advantage of the willingness of Jacksonville to explore new technologies that could play a key role in enhancing efficiency of the Jacksonville practice.
- The Task Force did not recommend a particular vendor at the time.

A few weeks following the meeting of the Board of Governors, Dr. Black walked into my office carrying a cup of coffee and sat down in one of my side chairs. When Dr. Black had questions about systems or technology, he would frequently drop by unannounced.

On this particular morning, the topic was on what to do next. He was persuaded that we should go to the next step in planning to attempt the paperless practice of medicine. He wanted to put together a steering group to guide the effort to work on vendor evaluation and transformation (transition) of the practice from paper-based to paperless, with a physician champion to work with me as the administrator in all aspects of the planning. I was confident that I could work with the physician he recommended for that role.

The program of Operation Efficiency at St. Luke's Hospital a year earlier had produced positive results to the bottom line with reduced expenses, staffing, and improved efficiencies. As the chair of the Hospital board, Dr. Black decided to engage the same consultants to conduct an Operation Efficiency program that would include both operation efficiency and the electronic medical record.

He shared the organization chart he had prepared. First was an oversight task force co-chaired by Dr. Black, Mr. Carleton Rider (chief administrative officer), and me. There were two task forces reporting to the oversight group. One was for the electronic medical record, which was chaired by my physician partner, with several other physicians and myself as the administrative support for the group. The other task force was for Operation Efficiency and was co-chaired by Dr. Black and Mr. Rider, with several physicians, including my physician partner, Mr. Harold Huber, COO, and myself as administrative support. Soon after our meeting, the Board of Governors approved his plan.

With our charge and team appointed, we spent much of that fall identifying the top three vendors from all of those we had visited. The three finalists included PHAMIS software, Cerner Corporation, and GTE. The first two companies had established software products; however, their primary healthcare applications were designed for hospitals, not the outpatient clinical settings. GTE did not have a product but wanted to collaborate with Mayo Clinic Jacksonville to design and build a product from the ground up.

The team preferred to start with an existing product suite and then modify or enhance it for use in our large integrated group practice. GTE was quickly eliminated from further consideration.

Mr. David Bolling, chief financial officer, advised us to avoid stating a preference for either of the two remaining companies. This was an excellent suggestion, because once we declared a choice, we would lose any bargaining power with the vendor.

By December 1993 Systems and Procedures was asked to revisit the staffing projection from the previous year. The Clinic had continued to add consulting staff, and the medical education program had grown over the intervening year. We made our rounds and updated the count of full-time equivalents. The number of people employed in these areas had grown to approximately 255. What would be the impact of the added growth during that year?

We had gathered a lot of information around our proposal, but we needed a detailed plan with the new capital requirements and ongoing maintenance costs, space requirements, and blueprints for networking all of the exam rooms. How could we modify the exam rooms to support a computer with a large monitor on the desk? Mr. Bolling and his team stepped in to help us develop of a pro forma.

CHAPTER NINE

Building the Pro Forma

A bank is a place that will lend you money
if you can prove that you don't need it.

—Bob Hope

There is a saying that when you approach a bank for a loan, the loan officer wants to see proof of your ability to repay the loan, such that you begin to doubt that you need the loan in the first place. Similarly, our proposal had far-reaching implications that would require significant capital investments, so we had to prove that our proposal would use the capital to produce savings in excess of the money we sought.

The savings had to pay back the capital investments plus the equivalent of interest on the money. At Dr. Black's request, Mr. Bolling took on the task of building a pro forma, which is a hypothetical financial picture based on previous business operations, for estimating the financial outcome of the automation.

Early on at Mayo Clinic, Systems and Procedures worked with Financial Analysis to develop proposals in which the capital costs were depreciated over the expected useful life of the assets. We expected a return on investment (ROI) over the stipulated useful life of the assets in the minimum range of 7 to 10 percent. Anything less was not likely to be approved. The greater the return, the more attractive the project was from a financial perspective; however, there were many other factors that could figure into the relative attractiveness of the proposal. We postulated that we could achieve significant staffing reductions through automation of the clinical practice. It was a complex proposal, and building a financial model that took into consideration all of the financial effects could help build our case and help with get the approvals necessary to invest the capital required.

Our team started building a list of what was needed. The list included an expanded data center to house the computing equipment, with potential space to grow as the equipment grew to meet the operational requirements. When the Davis Building was constructed, there was no need to include network wiring for each of the exam rooms, network closets, space for distributed network hubs and routers, or wiring sufficient for high availability of the computer workstations.

There were serious doubts about the clinical desk in every exam room, and the space to add a computer, mouse, keyboard, and twenty-one-inch monitor. We had to consider electrical and chiller capacity needed for the data center. The existing data center was located on the ground floor of the Davis Building, in the space that is now occupied by the pharmacy. It was constrained on all sides by other patient or administrative space, so growth in that location was not going to happen. We would need to build a new data center for the expanded computing capability, and construction costs had to be considered in the capital expenditures.

We contacted the potential software partners and requested estimates of the capital costs for lease or purchase of the hardware, licensing of the software, and ongoing operating expenses for software maintenance and upgrades. As we built the pro forma, the notion of conducting a pilot emerged. The paperless practice of medicine to increase efficiency of the physician and reduce expenses had never been done before.

The team settled on a six-month pilot period to test whether physicians could successfully practice medicine without needing the paper-based Plummer record, the professional service charge sheets (paper PSCs), or the Medical Service Requisition (paper-based ordering booklet) for ordering tests and consults. We believed six months was ample time to try the technology, stop and remediate any problems that surfaced, and then make another attempt. The leasing option stood out, because if we failed miserably, we could revert to the paper-based process easily. Leasing the software didn't bind us to a long-term commitment with unproven technology.

The first section of the pro forma listed the project capital for computer hardware, software, and data center construction for the first three years, beginning with 1993. Those same assets would begin depreciating in 1995, spreading them out over eight years, ending in 2002.

Next came the projected increases in operating expenses for hardware and software maintenance, other computer expenses for revenue cycle on a separate system, data center operations, networks and workstations, and additional information technology staffing for the same time period.

The next section of the pro forma projected the savings from salaries and benefits for the number of employees eliminated from the operational expense base. A sensitivity analysis was listed next, with eighty FTEs over eight years, with forty eliminated in the first year. The second bracket showed one hundred FTEs, with fifty eliminated in the first year. The third bracket showed one hundred twenty FTEs, with sixty eliminated in the first year. And finally, the last bracket showed one hundred forty FTEs, with seventy eliminated in the first year.

The break-even point in FTEs was calculated for each year, with sixty-five in 1995, and an overall average of seventy-two FTEs in the pro forma. Our projected FTEs at that time were in the range of 150 to 175, with a base of 255 FTEs in the areas that would be affected by elimination of the paper processes. If we were successful, we could easily produce a favorable return on the capital investment, but the *if*, was a very big if at the time.

When Mr. Bolling shared the first draft of the pro forma with Dr. Black and me, we were very pleased, and I felt that my original idea from years earlier was gaining traction. It was an exhilarating feeling, but the news was so good we could hardly believe our eyes. We walked through the numbers and, try as we might, could not find any flaws or errors.

Other factors had a dramatic impact on the return on investment that never went into the pro forma. When the project began, we operated an in-house print shop to produce many of the paper forms that went into the paper-based processes for the clinic. A large space in the warehouse was reserved to store and catalogue those 350 forms kept in inventory.

Prime clinical space in the Davis Building was occupied by medical records on the ground floor, with a lift system circulating buckets to carry the records and X-rays up to the clinical floors and gravity chutes to slide them back for archival storage.

General Services drove vans between facilities to transport medical records, X-rays, and laboratory specimens to the various outpatient clinical and inpatient hospital facilities.

The original Davis Building was four stories when I began working there in 1990. The rapid growth of patients, and the need to have more specialists and sub-specialists to build a large integrated group practice like the original in Rochester, Minnesota, drove the need to build additional floors. During my first two years in Jacksonville, the building grew to eight stories, and there was a horizontal expansion on the north side of the building mostly dedicated to administrative space initially.

The new sixth floor was built with half of the space dedicated to gastroenterology outpatient surgery. This configuration meant the Mayo Clinic could charge a facility fee for the GI procedures same as a hospital can, but ironically the State of Florida required these procedures to have a separate medical record distinct from the Plummer paper record, just at the time we were trying to automate the medical record.

When the group planned the addition, they anticipated growth over the following few years by building out some shelled-in space, but not finished into rooms and corridors. The other half of the sixth floor would become future exam rooms and physician offices, with desks built for the new computer configuration.

In the open space, a mock-up of the physician's desk and patient sofa was set up and tested for usability. One of the dilemmas was monitor placement. Prior rules dictated the patient could not see his medical record, which would put the monitor in the line of sight between the physician and the patient. Some physicians wanted to break with the rule and place the where it could be turned towards the patient to see her own medical information.

Some physicians preferred one side or the opposite, with no single setting that satisfied everyone. Based on that mock-up, the building design of that side of the floor was finalized and designated as the pilot area for the first attempt at the paperless practice of medicine. My physician partner's specialty was nephrology and hypertension, and he would be the first to attempt the paperless practice.

The pro forma and plan were beginning to take shape, and things seemed favorable, but we didn't have anything until we got approval from the Board of Governors and had endorsements from our physicians. Then there was the capital required. The list seemed to go on endlessly. Would we be able to get a favorable decision from the Board? What about the Mayo Clinic Group Practice Board and the Mayo Clinic Trustees? We still had a long way to go.

CHAPTER TEN

Spaghetti and Decisions

Quick decisions are unsafe decisions.

—Sophocles

As the year drew to a close, Dr. Black began to talk about a special meeting to make a decision regarding the proposed attempt to take the practice paperless. Dr. Black had a favorite meal in the staff cafeteria: spaghetti with meatballs, salad, and breadsticks. Everyone knew what he meant when he said, "Very soon we are going to have a spaghetti dinner and thoroughly discuss what we are going to do!"

The field of vendors had been narrowed to PHAMIS from Seattle and Cerner from Kansas City. I wanted an indepth assessment of both companies from the technical team. I assembled a group with representatives from data center operations, networking, programming, systems administrators, workstation support, database administration, and computer interfacing. This team was asked to do a comprehensive analysis of both organizations, to examine how the program code and libraries were managed, and how the systems were configured. The vendors would answer any questions from the Mayo Clinic team. An honest assessment of the information architecture, which was the technical underpinning for the respective systems, was needed for a clear recommendation.

The other question was how the proposed system would fit in with the other computer systems already in use at Mayo Clinic Jacksonville and St. Luke's Hospital. They had a week with each vendor to probe and get answers. After visits with both organizations, the team would make a recommendation of one vendor over the other, explaining the basis for their decision and the differences driving their recommendation. The team deliberations were completed by mid-December.

Meanwhile the Mayo Foundation Electronic Medical Record Planning Task Force had been meeting concurrently. The timing of the release of the report seemed to be intended to converge with the Jacksonville decision making.

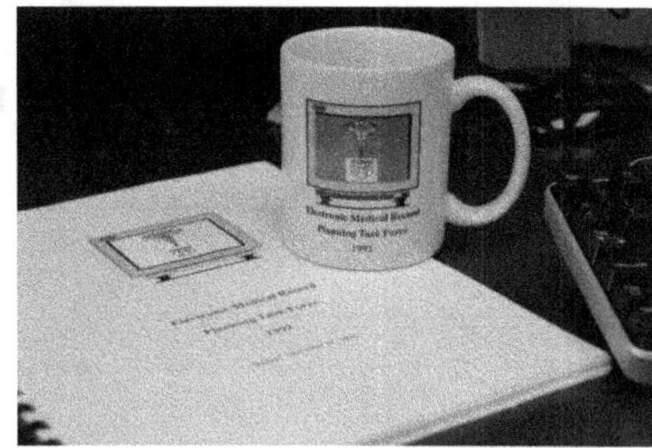

Report and comemorative mug are pictured here. Used with permission of Mayo Foundation for Medical Education and Research, all rights reserved.

There is an important distinction between what was viewed as an electronic medical record project by the Mayo Foundation Electronic Medical Record Planning Task Force and Jacksonville's quest for the automation of the clinical practice. The practice in Minnesota had many systems involved in its operations, including scheduling, ordering, billing, and registration systems, to name a few. They had several data centers and a large technical staff to build and maintain all of their systems.

By comparison, Mayo Clinic Jacksonville and St. Luke's Hospital each had a small data center, running turnkey systems, with very limited feature sets. Telecommunications were not nearly as advanced to the state of the technology that exists now for connecting between Florida and Minnesota. When the Jacksonville practice opened, the Information Services leadership in Rochester felt that they were not equipped with the technology or resources to support the new practice twelve hundred miles away in Jacksonville. A turnkey practice management system by CyCare provided the automation for the Clinic when I joined the staff.

St. Luke's ran on Shared Medical Systems (SMS), a service provider located in Malvern, Pennsylvania. The hospital laboratory ran Cerner, and Sunquest was the lab provider at the Clinic. Most other applications were microcomputer- or server-based.

The scope for what would be attempted in Jacksonville was to use an integrated architecture to automate scheduling, pharmacy, laboratory, electronic results viewing, and charging system. The results for financial purposes would be interfaced to CyCare for billing. In building this comprehensive automated system, we would attempt to eliminate the paper-based processes of scheduling, ordering, and charging, with an electronic medical record for viewing results. The other key component was the method we proposed physicians use to create their notes for the new medical record. A discussion of that process will be the subject of another chapter in this book.

On Tuesday, January 26, 1993, at 5:30 p.m., the members of the task force, the Board of Governors, and a representative from the Rochester Information Technology Department gathered in the staff dining room for the spaghetti supper Dr. Black had scheduled. (The representative from Rochester had also served on the Mayo Foundation Electronic Medical Record Planning Task Force.)

After eating, Dr. Black asked each group member for his or her recommendation for action, preferred vendor and why. Mr. Bolling reminded everyone that we would not announce our preferred vendor yet, deferring a definite decision. Everyone agreed to keep our choice a secret while the terms of the contract were negotiated and finalized. If we came to an impasse, we had the option of working with our second choice.

Several other issues were discussed that evening as goals were presented. First, we outlined the various steps going forward. We needed enough equipment and software to conduct the pilot program. We weren't sure of the readiness of the software application suites to support the paperless practice of medicine. The two final vendors had a number of hospital-based clients, but neither had done much work with outpatient practices, let alone large multi-specialty-based outpatient practices. Sufficient space to house the computer equipment and operations was a critical need to be addressed.

Since our technology partner would likely develop new software for us, we discussed the nature of the relationship, particularly in regards to the intellectual property. This would be an important issue in the contract negotiations.

Given the space on the sixth floor, the Board of Governors later settled which physician groups would be in the pilot group. They needed to time the pilot launch around completing the construction of the exam rooms and office space on the sixth floor and the new data center on the fifth floor.

The telephone switch for the original campus was on that floor, and the location of the point of presence for the network was housed there as well. We would need space for wiring closets on each of the floors. The closets would house the network hubs and routers needed for communication to the workstations in physician offices, secretarial workstations, exam rooms, and the desk areas. The exam rooms needed to be wired and the connections routed back to the wiring closets on each wing of the floor. Also the wiring closets needed to have uninterruptable power supplies and be connected to the campus generators in the event of loss of electrical service.

When the Clinic was built on the Davis property on the southeast corner of Duval County/Jacksonville, city water and sewer services had to be extended to the property, which was an expensive proposition. Due to the remote location when the practice opened in 1986, it was not uncommon for a passing thunderstorm to knock out power to the property. On at least one occasion, we lost our water service and had to close the practice for the day.

Running in a paperless mode on workstations, connected over networks to our new data center, had to be engineered carefully. The same was true for proposing to put a patient's medical record online and then not circulating the paper record. What would happen when a thunderstorm knocked out the power in the middle of the afternoon?

Besides the challenges of the organization, we had environmental issues, utility redundancy, and administrative challenges. Then the issue of converting physicians from using the nearly one-hundred-year-old Plummer paper record to one on a computer workstation. What was to become of us as we took on these challenges?

CHAPTER ELEVEN

Dictation and Transcription

Writer's cramp was God's gift to clinical notes.

—Leo F. Black, M.D.

Automating the clinical practice and moving to a computer-based medical record raised several substantial issues, such as:

- Most physicians never learned to type, and had not been expected to typewrite their clinical notes;
- Physician time was too valuable to be wasted on clerical tasks that required extensive keyboard entry;
- Any process that could not be completed quickly and easily, like handwritten notes, would introduce additional delay in the movement of the medical record; and
- Changing the process from handwritten to electronic notes would require a cultural change for the typical Mayo Clinic consultant.

Finally, there is a general perception that most physician handwriting is illegible, or nearly so.

As Systems and Procedures went about their work in examining increasing the efficiency for the practice, it was observed at the time that when a new consultant joined the staff, typically, they requested and received approval to hire a desk attendant and secretary. It was a generally accepted practice that each physician would need at least this much assistance in completing his or her day-to-day work. The result was that the allied health staff was growing much faster than the consultants were.

This model had to change if Mayo Clinic Jacksonville was going to reduce operating overhead and become more efficient, but the administrative staff knew it would be a delicate challenge to break the pattern. The physician leadership knew we had to build a new model for meeting the secretarial needs of the physician. By converting to a computer-based medical record, the desk staffing could be drastically reduced but that was only one part of the problem. Changing the secretarial model was another important part of the equation that had to be addressed.

Anticipating the need to keep physicians efficient and find new ways to build clinical notes, we looked at introducing dictation and transcription as the relatively easy to use, new way to get clinical information into the electronic medical record. But adding transcriptionists without changing the medical secretary model would not solve the problem either.

With the support of our physician leaders, we began to look at our existing dictation and transcription systems, with a view toward how things needed to function with this replacement process and the subsequent process model. The turnaround time for dictated and transcribed clinical notes would become a critical factor. Ms. Rachel Martin from Systems and Procedures took charge of reengineering the secretarial work into two distinct roles. The first was to continue with the conventional medical secretary position, but with a higher ratio of the number of physicians covered.

The other was the full-time transcriptionist role. Transcriptionists would work in pools, with a clearly defined work list to be transcribed, and any given job for a clinical note would go to the next available transcriptionist. Rachel's work was outstanding, and over time we changed the culture to move from one secretary dedicated to work with one physician to becoming a shared resource serving three or more physicians, depending on the workload.

In discussions with the potential technology partners, it was clear we would require a large-scale dictation and transcription platform since hundreds of clinical notes would be created every day, with correspondence to referring physicians and patients. Part of the traditional Mayo Clinic product after receiving an evaluation from a physician is a final letter to the patient regarding the doctor's findings, and to the referring physician if the patient has been seen in response to a referral. The transcription process would not only produce the clinical note but also create draft correspondence from the final clinical note.

Our ideal vision was that when the physician completed the patient visit, he would click a button on the computer screen. The automated system would take note of the patient appointment, collecting the appointment type, the identity of the patient, and the physician seeing the patient. In doing that, the computer would capture the critical information for indexing and filing the clinical note. With this information, the computer system would call the physician on her pager and notify her that the system was ready to receive the dictation.

All of the typical dictation features would be available, for example, pause, edit, rewind, and playback of the digitized voice recording, using the number button keys on the phone for control. The completed dictation would go to a work queue for a transcription pool of waiting work, where the next available transcriptionist would select and complete the transcription process.

When the draft note was transcribed, it would be picked up by the electronic medical record system, and the doctor would receive notification that the draft document was ready for review and finalization. The draft would also be labeled as such but made available for the rest of the practice, so the next physician seeing the patient would have the findings available. Some delay is created, but we felt with this new model, the turnaround time would be no greater than the total elapsed time with the handwritten notes and movement of the paper charts.

When the physician saw her draft note for the first time, it might be complete and accurate. If not, the physician had an opportunity to make corrections or revisions, and the revised note would be available in the electronic record. The software would now display the corrected note. A physician who had seen and treated the patient based on an earlier version of the note would be able to see the previous note thanks to a software feature called versioning. Versioning keeps the most recent version of a note plus any prior versions. Physicians who may have treated a patient on an earlier version would receive a message that the note they had based clinical decisions on had been changed by the author, which might have an impact on how they were treating the patient.

Cerner identified the Sudbury Systems Corporation as one of the leading companies at the time that was compatible with their architecture. The Sudbury system consisted of a Digital Equipment Corporation (DEC) PDP-11 with software linking it to a telephone system. We believed we could develop the interfacing just described. As an interim step, we connected the system to our phone system with group of trunk lines to the switch.

A physician would dial the dictation system using any phone, key in his identification (a five-digit number), and be prompted for the patient medical record and a work type for the note indexing and priority. Professional transcriptionists would see a prioritized list of physician notes waiting to be transcribed. The waiting work was completed by priority.

For example, a clinical note on an active patient was a top priority. By comparison, a final note that generated the correspondence was a lower priority, since turnaround time was not as critical.

The other part of this process was collecting all of the transcribed notes on a server so the electronic medical record computer system could periodically interrogate the server, picking up the new work to be indexed and integrated into the medical record without needless duplication. Typically the EMR system would interrogate the server every minute or so, such that the EMR was current regarding clinical findings for a given patient.

In August of 1993, the transcription server was available to begin collecting dictated clinical notes, but we didn't have the Sudbury System available yet, so we used what was referred to as "sneaker net." Doctors getting their first start with dictations used little voice recorders, dictating their notes and then putting the tape cassettes in the envelope with the paper-based medical record. It was a makeshift process, and we had a number of misplaced cassettes, lost cassettes, and notes attributed to the wrong patients, all of which created huge problems with the process and threatened the survival of the shift to dictation.

But the immediate significant benefit the physicians saw was that the clinical notes were clearly legible now, much clearer than the handwritten versions.

Another change: Secretarial coverage ratios began to shift. A physician's work no longer required a dedicated secretary. We converted building space into transcription work areas on each floor. This nearby physical location enabled the physician to make corrections on her clinical notes and correspondence.

The location of the transcription workrooms became a problem for transcription productivity, though. A transcriptionist works best when he can do straight transcribing without interruption. By being located physically close to the desk on each floor, it was impossible for a transcriptionist to receive productivity incentives.

This is an example of a dictation sent to a transcriptionist by one of the physicians who was learning to use the dictation process. (The names have been changed to protect the identity of the parties involved.)

> Letter to Dr. John Brown with copy to Dr. Abe Cohen, including first extensive dictation on 12-7-93. But, of course, you will not include the sentence that says I will see Mrs. Newman after she is seen by Dr. Monroe, neurologist, and by Dr. Miller, orthopedic surgeon. Forget that sentence, eliminate it from the letter. Put the paragraphs about Dr. Monroe's and Dr. Mil-

> ler's visit right up above the last paragraph which says "Mrs. Newman is in a period of her life where she has episodic crying spells." Make a paragraph after that sentence, or just before, or make a new paragraph where it says I also reviewed with Mrs. Newman her consults with Dr. Monroe and another new paragraph where it starts with Dr. Williams, gynecologist, and then make another paragraph where it says, excuse me, forget that last sentence where it says that she is willing to start insulin, or transfer that sentence where she says that she is willing to start the insulin after she has seen Dr. John Brown and we will write him—transfer that to the sentence where it says, where it talks about a combination of NPH and regular will be necessary and then put Mrs. Newman is will to start insulin after she has seen and then in the letter to Dr. Brown just put you, not the rest of that sentence. That's about it. Thanks.

It took the transcriptionist more than two hours to complete these instructions. It would take time to complete the shift to transcriptionists, but we were riding a learning curve, and the transformation from handwritten notes to transcribed was well underway.

Another technology attempt was to use a "quick key" system that would notice frequently used phrases or acronyms and explode it into the full phrase. An example would be CABG (pronounced cabbage), when typed in the transcription model, it would expand into the full phrase "coronary artery bypass and graft," thereby increasing a transcriptionists efficiency. One of the early notes that gave us all (except for Dr. Black) a laugh, exploded a phrase with the keyword of black into "Dr. Black tarry stool." That error in the system was quickly corrected.

When the prototype electronic medical record was established, we performed a *back file conversion* from those early servers into the database that became the first repository of the clinical notes created by the dictation/transcription process. The term back file conversion can refer to many things, but in the sense used in this book simply, it means taking medical record documents captured before the emergence of the EMR and identifying the means for how they would be handled in the paperless environment.

For example, handwritten notes at Mayo Clinic date back to 1907, when the first Plummer medical record was put into use. In the system we used, our means for handling that paper record in the paperless environment was by scanning and indexing each page of the documents, using the same structure for the Plummer medical record. As we automated, more and more of the record material on a patient would be captured and presented in electronic form, and eventually the need to scan paper documents would disappear.

Since the transcribed note was much more readable, it could always be used in the paper-based medical record as long as it was being circulated. We were learning how to capture clinical notes efficiently and how to get them into the electronic medical record effectively. That was the first wave of cultural change introduced in the plan to go paperless. The next hurdle was for the physicians to accept and use the EMR. Could we get them to the point of preferring it over the paper-based medical record? We felt like we were in a delicate and precarious place, and only time would tell the outcome.

CHAPTER TWELVE

Imaging and MegaSars

Any sufficiently advanced technology is indistinguishable from magic.

—Arthur C. Clarke

Dictation and transcription of new data was just one of the many steps in fully transitioning to EMR. It was essential to convert images of the paper documents in the medical record too.

In the world of the paper-based medical records, the competition to get the single medical record by those involved in caring for the patient was enormous. It was essential to see a comprehensive summary of everything being done in connection with the care of the patient so that appropriate decisions could be made about next steps in their care.

When we looked at patient records, they ranged from new patients with no previous record at Mayo Clinic to long-term patients. For the prior, we aimed to capture as much information as we could electronically so the bulk of their record would be electronic. Unfortunately, until the entire outpatient practice had embraced the EMR, we would have to circulate the paper record, creating a dual record system. That was the worst possible option for health care, creating the potential question of which was the accurate chart, the paper or the computer record.

A physician resisting the pressure to use the computer could throw up the argument that the computer did not have everything that was in the paper record; therefore, physicians needed both, although realistically, they did not have time to review everything in both records. This caused us to create one of the first principles: both records had to be complete. So we had allied health staff perform quality checks on both records to ensure they were in complete agreement before being given to the physician.

Skeptical physicians would play a game I dubbed "Stump the Computer." A physician who was getting ready to see patients with the EMR would take a paper chart and do a side-by-side comparison of the paper record with that on the computer. Were they to find something in the paper chart that was not in the computer, they would report the discrepancy with glee and return to the familiar paper record for that patient encounter. Discrepancies were extremely rare and, we had a technical team ready to remediate the situation if one occurred.

When we started working on this project, imaging technology had been successfully implemented in other industries, eliminating many file cabinets and freeing up expensive storage space. And access to archived files improved the efficiencies for the staff needing to refer to the stored records. The most expensive part of the technology was online storage, which used spinning disk arrays.

An Atlanta-based company, IMNET Systems, had developed some innovative technology for building huge archives of records. Mayo Clinic Jacksonville had nearly a half million medical records at the planning stage of this project. We had metal storage shelves from floor to ceiling filled with medical records. Previous operational studies revealed that typically less than 30 percent of the charts are active at any given time. The bulk of the records sat on the shelves until a patient returned for a visit. Based on this information, we projected how many records might be active at any given time and estimated the amount of disk storage required to keep just the active charts on the more expensive magnetic disks.

The IMNET technology required us to microfilm our medical records pages, with the production negative kept in an off-site archival storage facility. We would have two positive copies, one would be kept in an on-campus storage facility, and the other copy would be loaded into a MegaSar. The MegaSar had the microfilm projector on the top of a large metal cabinet that housed several hundred microfilm cassettes. A sample of the microfilm cassette is shown here with the film leader.

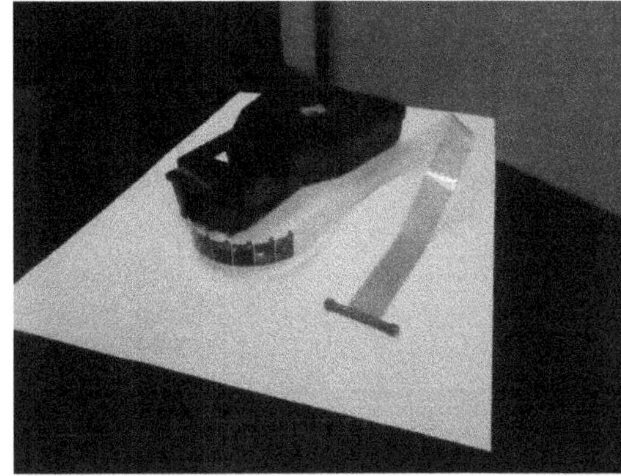

The plan was for the automated system to produce a list of patients who had appointments for the next day. In anticipation of a patient arriving for an appointment, the computer system would make a request for the images of the paper medical record, find the appropriate cassette(s) on the MegaSar, locate the associated frames, and capture the images to the magnetic storage.

When the physician saw the patient the next day, they could see the patient record with data captured electronically, or images of the paper chart. The important thing was that the full paper chart did not need to be retrieved and delivered to the physician. More importantly, others involved in care for the same patient could access the information simultaneously, without having to wait for the paper record.

Just as we were working on getting this technology planned for our project, several other forces were at work, forcing us to reconsider some things.

The first was what I characterized as the time decay of medical information. The more timely the information, the better, and the older the information, the less useful. For example, if a physician discovers that the patient has hypertension, recommendations and medications are used to manage the patient's blood pressure. Once under control, hypertension becomes less of an issue since the patient is taking medication, and possibly implementing other diet and/or lifestyle modifications, to help manage the symptoms.

When my physician partner saw the size of some of the charts that needed to be imaged, he balked at the amount of labor necessary to complete the task, so he suggested an alternative plan. Just scan the most recent history and physical, radiology results, laboratory results, and other diagnostic tests.

We were looking for ways to be more efficient, so we tried his suggestion. The result was that we now had to look at each page for date, type of result, and then parcel them out into a separate packet, scan them, and then reassemble the medical record back into the customary structure. That process was compared with simply taking the entire medical record and scanning it all at once. It was actually faster to convert the entire record, rather than to select out the most recent results. Plus we ran the risk of a physician finding out about a major medical procedure that had been completed successfully years earlier, who would then call for the paper record if the procedure wasn't considered recent enough to include with the more recent brief edition.

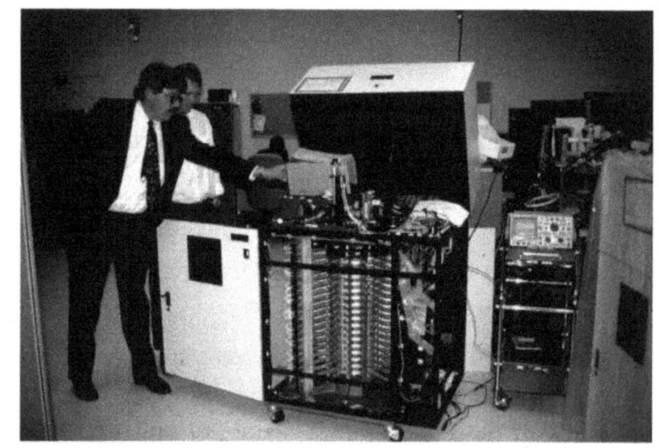

MegaSar at the production facility ready to be shipped. A fully loaded MegaSar could hold millions of images on microfilm.

Mr. W. Jeff Smith (no relation), who reported to me, was the technologist working with the MegaSar technology. Jeff had an excellent technical background and years of experience that matched or exceeded most of his peers in IT. The technology, while it looked promising, was not working well enough for a production system, and the problems we experienced with the MegaSar were burning him out. He finally came to me and said there had to be a better way to solve the problem.

Jeff had observed that a recent breakthrough with miniaturization had caused the price of magnetic storage to drop precipitously. He did some calculations, looking at the expense of the MegaSar technology, and compared it with what could be accomplished with RAID 5 technology. He concluded the MegaSar technology had become obsolete. He shared his analysis with me, and I was convinced of the merits of his suggestions. I called the CEO at IMNET and reported our findings. He listened and then asked for some time to talk with his leadership.

When he called back, he asked if he could send his CFO down to review our findings. When he arrived, we walked him through our analysis with the cost numbers, and he was a bit chagrined but admitted we were correct. He arranged for the MegaSars to be packed up and shipped back to Atlanta, and Mayo Clinic was credited with the return.

RAID 5 is an acronym for random array of inexpensive drives, and the suffix number is the highest in a sequence of zero to five. With this technology the files were distributed across many disk drives. Should one of the hard drives fail or crash, it could be pulled out of the array, with a new replacement drive inserted in its place. Shutting off the power to the array was not necessary for replacing the drive, and the software didn't require a reboot. The software for the array could look at the information on the other drives, and what was stored on each drive, then rebuild the contents on the offending drive when it failed. This was impressive technology at a competitive price, which emerged at just the right time for our project.

Keeping the images on RAID 5 storage greatly enhanced responsiveness for our clinical users and reduced some of the early grumbling about the computer being too slow. With dictation and transcription as the primary means of creating new clinical notes, imaging capable of converting the paper-based medical records, and the direct feeds of clinical results from the laboratory, we believed we had all of the key ingredients for the paperless practice of medicine.

The question loomed: How would we get these systems to work in harmony, in order to quit circulating the paper-based medical record altogether? What would we learn once a working prototype was in place?

CHAPTER THIRTEEN

The Prototype

You never change things by fighting the existing reality. To change something, build a new model that makes the existing model obsolete.

—R. Buckminster Fuller

We had agreed on our preferred systems vendor following the spaghetti supper. Mr. Bolling lead the negotiation team for Mayo Clinic, defining the terms of the contract. Our in-house counsel assisted him from the Legal Department, along with the director of the medical laboratory, and me. The lead from Cerner Corporation was a senior executive. We asked for the rights to use all of the relevant Cerner application software since we had no idea which components of the application suite might be needed to go paperless. As part of the contract, we tackled the thorny problem of intellectual property that might occur during the course of our project.

Mayo Clinic Jacksonville wasn't interested in developing programming code or in the attendant responsibilities for maintaining it. We wanted Cerner to manage those responsibilities, but we didn't want to have to license the right to software developed as a result of our collaboration. We settled on having a perpetual right to use the applications developed under our agreement. Dr. Black felt it fair to pay maintenance fees to ensure the code was properly maintained and compliant with all medical and legal requirements. The general feeling by local leadership was that development and maintenance of computer software was outside of our core business.

We negotiated the contract with Cerner and had it completed by the end of the first quarter of 1993. One of the requirements of the contract was for Cerner to build a prototype for those of us who were around the table for the spaghetti supper as soon as possible.

The clinical electronic medical record program created by Cerner uses the brand identification *PowerChart* for all clinical users. It contains all of the necessary communication elements for physicians to support the paperless practice of medicine. I believed the physicians needed to get familiar with PowerChart as soon as we could make it available in a comfortable environment, such as the privacy of their own offices. This proved to be an interesting component of gaining physician acceptance of the computer-based paperless practice.

The very first charts loaded on the system were mock-up records, which were useful for demonstrations and training. As networks were wired into additional physician offices, they were connected to the system so they had ample time to get familiar with the application and user interface in a nonthreatening environment.

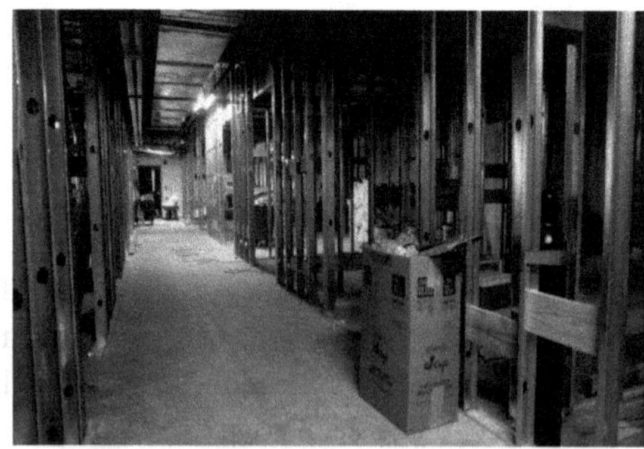

Construction of the space for the pilot on sixth floor
Used with permission of Mayo Foundation for Medical Education and Research, all rights reserved.

Construction on the buildout of the sixth floor for the exam rooms and offices was not due to be complete until December 1993. In the meanwhile, other items were in process. For example, facilities had contractors working on weekends and after hours wiring the rooms for network connections.

The physician chair of the Information Technology Committee in Rochester had the vision and foresight to sponsor a separate project to add a network infrastructure for the three major sites. He worked with the then IT administrator responsible for networks at the time, and he took a design and proposal to the Trustees for a large capital appropriation. The ethernet protocol would run on category 5 wires or fiber optic cabling, depending on the size and speed of the information being conveyed on the network.

We anticipated that if we began sending large radiographic images or visual images, we might need the speed possible with fiber optic cabling, so every exam room and office had wire pulled from the network closets, ready for the eventual rollout of the EMR throughout the facility. Optionally, with fiber optic-based network cards in the computers, they could be equipped to work on the fiber optic network at very high speeds if necessary.

Since no one had anticipated needing computer network capability previously, or the necessity for closets to house the network hubs and routers, we had to identify space to house the equipment and network connections in the Mayo buildings, and then we had to consider what would happen in the event of a power outage. Into this increasingly complex set of requirements, we needed uninterruptible power supplies, and the outlets needed to be powered with generators in the event of a power failure. Power outlets, which will work on emergency power in the health care setting, are typically colored red to connote the reliability for those situations.

Next on the list for consideration was what would happen if a network card failed. Hot swappable cards were used in the routers so if one failed, it could be pulled from the router and replaced without powering down all of the network connections on the floor. Loss of a floor with ten or more exam rooms would cripple the practice. We looked at some of the room utilization studies and determined that if the computer failed in an exam room, the physician and patient likely could move to the room next door or across the hall and work with the computer in that room while the failed workstation was put back in service. We were able to achieve this configuration by putting every fourth room on a different network segment.

Since those early days, networks have progressed with self-healing equipment, much higher speeds, new protocols, wireless capabilities, tighter security, and many improvements that have made them more resilient. The problems we experienced are now a rarity. A redundant fiber optic backbone was put in place, connecting all of the floors in the Davis Building, and eventually connecting buildings. With our location being relatively rural in those early days, our network lines between buildings were hit by lightning and vaporized on a couple of occasions, with the afternoon thunderstorms so common in Florida during the summers.

The connection between St. Luke's Hospital and Mayo Clinic Jacksonville was through leased lines from two different carriers so the circuits would be divergent. But an accident with a backhoe along San Pablo Road revealed the two carriers we used had their lines, the ones that gave us the divergent path, in the same trench, side by side. From then on the vendor had to demonstrate the actual routes for the wiring to assure the lines were truly divergent. In one case, we discovered the routes were divergent until they got to St. Luke's Hospital, and then again, the trench with the wires from the street up to the point of presence in the hospital had them side by side.

With the new data center on the fifth floor of the Davis Building, Cerner delivered the first VAX computer running Digital Equipment Corporation's (DEC) VMS operating system. The data repository was built with the Oracle relational database management system. This first system was configured to carry us through the six-month pilot period that began Tuesday, January 4, 1994.

Following the pilot, Cerner agreed to remedy any defects within six months. In the event of a total failure of the automation of the clinical practice using the Cerner system, it would be shut down, disassembled, and everything sent back. Our plan, as Dr. Black liked to say, in this case, would be to wait until Rochester delivered a system.

We anticipated that system availability would be an issue if not properly addressed. The machine room was elevated to facilitate wiring for the computer systems to be placed under the moveable floor panels. Two separate air conditioning systems were available to chill the space if the primary system failed. Power was provided by a huge uninterruptible power supply in addition to the utility power feed. This system would detect the slightest interruption and switch over to feed seamlessly so the users wouldn't notice a power failure.

A couple of years later, Facilities was able to configure power with the Jacksonville Electric Authority to feed the campus from two separate power grids, so if the primary grid failed, detection of the loss of one would switch the campus emergency power over to the other grid within fifteen seconds. We went to extraordinary lengths to make the system as reliable as possible. It was high availability for the system, but not fault tolerant.

At the same time the new data center was being constructed on the fifth floor of the Davis Building, Cerner was busily putting together the products to build the prototype called for in our contract, and we had to begin adding staff to support the Cerner system. Facilities worked on the blueprints and permits, followed by the actual construction of the exam rooms, physician offices, and secretarial space, all in short order.

We had settled on twenty-two-inch monitors since they were capable of reproducing a sheet of medical record information at the same size as the paper, thereby providing easily readable documents for our doctors.

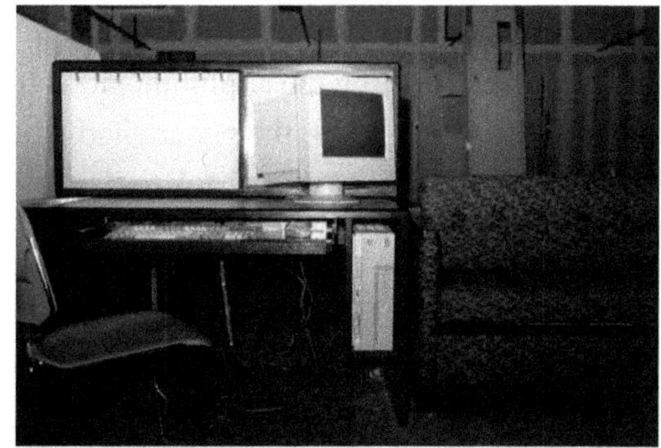

Mockup of the exam room configuration in the shelled in space.
Used with permission of Mayo Foundation for Medical Education and Research, all rights reserved.

The best way to resolve the question was to build a mock-up in the vacant shelled-in space so physicians could sit at the desk and see how it felt. We debated about putting an X-ray viewing box in the new exam rooms since most of the physicians assigned to the pilot space would not read their X-rays. The neurosurgeons would be the exception.

We wanted to equip each desk with a space where the computer with hard drive could be serviced easily, and then we needed a place for the keyboard and mouse. Space was constructed on the side of the knee space for the computer, and a pullout tray was built into the desk to accommodate the mouse and keyboard.

The PowerChart application at the time used Oracle for the database, and the application ran in a terminal emulation program called X-Windows. A photographic example of a test record in the prototype with the image of a paper record is shown here.

For the pilot, our scanning team would look for upcoming appointments and determine if the patient had been seen previously. If so, then the team member would locate the paper-based record and convert it with the imaging technology for the patient chart. Ideally, the paper record and the computer record would be in perfect harmony and available for the physician during the appointment. If there was a problem with the computer at any point, the paper chart was available for the physician, and she could always go back to paper to complete the appointment.

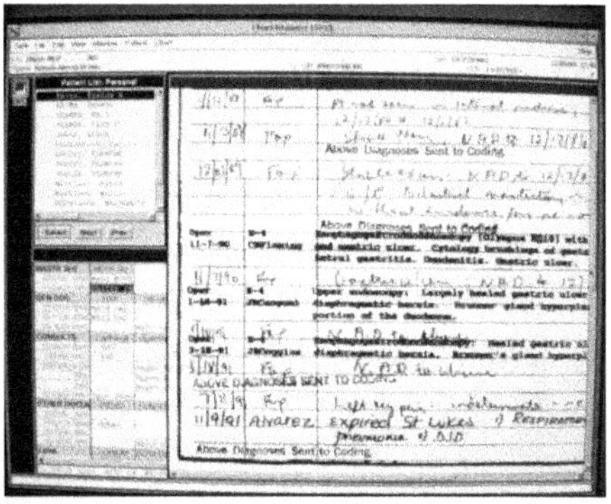

X-windows prototype with test data.
Used with permission of Mayo Foundation for Medical Education and Research, all rights reserved.

When we had the prototype complete and working, we felt ready to conduct the pilot. The next step was the readiness of the physician. Would it work for our doctors? Following the Christmas and New Year's holidays, the pilot would start. How would all of the work and planning turn out?

CHAPTER FOURTEEN

The Pilot

Before you become too entranced with gorgeous gadgets and mesmerizing video displays, let me remind you that information is not knowledge, knowledge is not wisdom, and wisdom is not foresight. Each grows out of the other, and we need them all.

—Arthur C. Clarke

My physician partner was the leader who planned to conduct the first paperless patient encounter on Tuesday, January 4, 1994, on one of his patients scheduled for the day. Mondays tended to be busy, with activities from the weekend rolling into the day, so he selected Tuesday as a better day to begin the experiment. The exam room was ready for the first paperless encounter. Room number 83 on the sixth floor, on the B-side of the desk, was used for the first attempt at a paperless patient encounter.

My physician partner appeared a bit shaken when he emerged from the exam room following that appointment. He said he had to "rewire" his brain, because the new process changed his whole way of thinking about how he conducted the appointment. He said the paper charts now felt almost like a prop when he walked into the exam room. If he reached a point where he was uncertain what to say next, he could take part of the paper results and discuss the contents with the patient. This time he walked into the room with hands empty, with only his stethoscope. He knew what he needed to say to the patient, brought up his medical record on the computer, and conducted the session. He said he completed a normal evaluation appointment in about forty-five minutes. That first paperless encounter took him nearly an hour and a half, but he completed it without calling for the paper record.

With the experience of that first encounter, we learned a physician inexperienced in using a computer-based record would need to have her schedule lightened while learning how to use the system. We established the principle that each physician would have a lighter schedule while adapting to the computer-based record. On average, they were up to speed with the computer within two weeks, reverting to their previous schedule of patients.

One of the physicians in the pilot group was Dr. John Mentel, who worked in the General Internal Medicine division. He was experienced in using a personal computer at home and was very computer literate. He had recently joined the Jacksonville practice from private practice, even though he had completed his residency at Mayo Clinic in Rochester. He made huge contributions to the completion of the automation project, from the pilot program on. He was always willing to serve in alpha testing of new products and applications. His feedback as we tried new technology products and innovations proved invaluable.

It did not take anywhere near the six-month pilot to know the Automated Clinical Practice was a success. It was clear before March. Most of the physicians on the B-side of the sixth floor had adapted to the paperless practice. We planned to omit paper-based records on that floor when all of the physicians were adept with using the new system. The staff, freed up by the reduced workload, were reassigned to the scanning and quality control area to ensure the paper and computer charts matched perfectly.

Almost immediately, the converts offered the following observation about improved efficiency: Before the EMR, a patient would call the office and ask to speak with her physician about a question on her medication or treatment plan. The secretary would have to write down the patient information, promise to call her back, request the location of the paper record, convey the record back to the physician so that he or she could review the information and question, and finally call the patient back to answer the question. After the EMR, doctors could answer a call and look up the information on the computer and answer the question immediately. They were so pleased with how the addition of the computer access to the patient record had made them so much more efficient and allowed them to provide a much higher level of care for their patients.

Insistence on putting the computer in the physicians' offices well in advance of going paperless paid off in big dividends. It provided time for them to become familiar with the computer-based record in a nonthreatening situation. No one likes to be embarrassed by making a mistake in front of others. A physician learning to operate the computer system could practice in the office without the pressure of trying to use the computer in front of patients.

We developed a sequence of events for getting physicians to use the computer for their paperless practices. First, they had to adapt to the use of dictation and transcription successfully. Next, they would work with their workstation in their offices, learning to use the system with confidence. When they felt ready to start their paperless encounters, we would shorten their schedule of appointments by an hour per day during the first two weeks. When they were past the learning curve, seeing patients with the computer chart and no paper record, they would signal that they were ready to resume their normal patient load.

Converting from handwritten notes to dictated and transcribed notes sounds simple and easy. Instead of writing, one simply took a voice recorder and spoke his or her notes, but we quickly learned it wasn't that simple for everyone. Dr. Black liked to remind us that writer's cramp is what kept paper-based clinical notes short and to the point. Physicians who had previously produced crisp and concise medical record notes, when given the opportunity for dictation, turned from being a Hemingway (brief and concise) to a Tolstoy (thorough and lengthy), some reaching as much as four single-spaced, typewritten sheets of transcribed content. While comprehensive, it was too much information, in too great of detail. My physician partner and other physician leaders would ask transcriptionists for names of colleagues who needed coaching about the length of their dictated clinical notes.

Another issue was the structure of the content of the note. For example, getting everyone to list the presenting complaint at the same place in the outline used, followed by such things as onset, symptoms, and family and social history, etc. was important. Well-organized templates had a big impact on each doctor's productivity. Our physician leaders worked with each department and division to build standard dictation templates. We recognized variation between specialties or subspecialties as appropriate, but we worked at length to achieve standardization and uniformity to improve physician efficiency in reading clinical notes throughout the practice.

And templates for different purposes had an important impact on transcriptionists and secretarial efficiency. For example, we developed a template for the return visit. This was the appointment when the physician sat down with the patient and reviewed all of the findings of the clinic visit. It included notes from other consults, lab results, radiology, and diagnostic tests. And the physician would share recommendations and a treatment plan with the patient.

Some education may be involved to teach the patient how to manage her disease. The note summarizing the return visit was completed for the patient and put in her medical record. We had a template that would take some portion of the note and make it available to the doctor's medical secretary for use in the letter to the referring physician and to the patient, both of whom were very important to the practice. This feature saved the physicians time by eliminating the dictation part of the letter, which would contain much of the same content.

Templates were developed for general evaluations (EVAL), comprehensive history and physicals (CHP), specialty consults (CONS), and so on. Surgery and Radiology had long used dictation and transcription for capturing the notes for surgical procedures. Radiology used a very efficient system referred to as direct dictation.

Even though the benefits of EMR were becoming obvious, not all of the physicians immediately embraced the paperless practice of medicine. Everett Rogers argues that the *diffusion of innovations* is the process by which an innovation is communicated through certain channels over time, among the participants in a social system.[1] With successive groups adopting the new technology, there are innovators, early adopters, early majority, late majority, and finally, laggards. Those groups were consistent with our observations.

The Internet was in its infancy in the early 1990s, and the minority of homes in the United States had computers, and typically the number of users in the family was very small or singular. Physicians in our practice who used a computer at home adapted very quickly to the new practice environment. The physicians with no computer in the home had a much bigger hurdle. Typically they had no experience with a keyboard or touch typing, so they had to use "hunt and peck" typing, a tedious process.

Many physicians today regard any tasks requiring use of a keyboard as "clerical" work. As an alternative method, we used the Windows features with selection lists and the mouse for point-and-click entry as much as possible to avoid a physician having to use the keyboard.

I recall arriving at work in my office early one morning during the pilot period to find that one of my physician colleagues had carefully photocopied an article from a professional journal about a practice from another part of the country where an attempt to computerize the practice had failed miserably. The part of the article citing the failure was highlighted in neon yellow, and the message did not have any identification on it whatsoever. The project was getting good reviews with some parts pf the practice, but in other parts, the laggards were secretly hoping the pilot would fail and the computers would go away.

The support from Dr. Black and the Board of Governors was outstanding. I recall Dr. Black told me, "Reg, as you work on the

---

[1] Everett M. Rogers, *Diffusion of Innovations* (Glencoe: Free Press, 1962), p. 22.

automation of the clinical practice, you may encounter a physician who will tell you that you cannot do something. You tell them that they need to come and talk with me about it."

He recognized the need for the practice to become more efficient and gave me his full and unflinching support. It was not a license to ride roughshod over the staff, but a sign that if there was a good reason to do a part of the automation to meet the needs of the practice, I had his support. In getting approval for our project from the governing bodies, Dr. Black argued successfully that all three Mayo Clinic sites could work independently at automation since it required innovative technology applications and had not been accomplished successfully at the time.

Still, the physicians who tried the paperless practice and achieved a few successful encounters created a buzz in the staff cafeteria at lunch. The stories—like taking a call from a patient and being able to answer the question while they were still on the phone—were positive, and we were getting good reviews from our physician users.

The pilot had started, and seemed successful, but could we get all the physicians to embrace the technology? We had a lot to learn.

CHAPTER FIFTEEN

Growing the Pilot to Production

If it keeps up, man will atrophy all his limbs but the push-button finger.

—Frank Lloyd Wright

Once the pilot started, there was no turning back. Typically at the end of a pilot period, an organization would shut down the system and perform a thorough evaluation of the findings about the successes, weaknesses, things to be improved upon, perhaps some system remediation, and then they would decide the outcome and benefits achieved. That never happened with our pilot.

Once the physicians worked with the computer-based record, they were not willing to allow any outages at all, for any reason. With the Cerner system, maintenance on the files was scheduled to occur after midnight on Tuesday, and again at midnight on Saturday.

We were working with a performance standard of high availability, not fault-tolerant, which means the system was available in the range of 95 to 98 percent. The following table shows examples of availability based upon total days per year, hours per month, and hours per week. The Cerner system as a high availability system ran in the 97 to 98 percent range or higher by my observation over the years.

Availability	Downtime per year	Downtime per month	Downtime per week
90%	36.5 days	72 hours	16.8 hours
95%	18.25 days	36 hours	8.4 hours
97%	10.96 days	21.6 hours	5.04 hours
98%	7.30 days	14.4 hours	3.36 hours

By comparison, a fault tolerant system was designed to never go down or fail, giving the users 100 percent availability. Typically everything is redundant from the data center, through the network. To have fault tolerant performance in the exam room, every room would need to have two computer workstations, each fed by a separate network all the way back to the main computer system, thereby eliminating any single point of failure. The expense associated with this fault tolerant system was quite a bit higher than the high availability configuration. The physician leadership felt the practice would find high availability adequate when balanced against the added cost of configuring for a fault tolerant operation.

Once our physicians embraced the technology, they would have preferred the fault tolerant approach, but that was not financially feasible. The point: The physicians loved the system once they had adapted to it! There was no more talk in the staff cafeteria about getting rid of the automated clinical practice. Now people were talking about the rollout and some of the growing pains we experienced.

During the pilot period, we maintained a dual record system. Part of the system operations was still running the former paper-based system, which included the Plummer medical record, the MSR charge sheets for ordering and scheduling, and the PSC paper-based charge sheets. All of these components were now operating on the automated clinical practice, too, where we had physicians in physical areas of the outpatient building. In the medical practice setting, a dual record system is the most difficult process of all, because of the duplication of effort in keeping both the paper and electronic records synchronized. The technology was working, but the number of documents being stored on the system and the number of users was growing. The growth resulted in slowed system response at peak times.

We had anticipated the need for additional capital to grow the system. Dr. Black had planned to report on the pilot at the August meeting of the Mayo Clinic Board of Trustees. With the success of the program, we demonstrated the system to the president of the American Medical Association that April, and Dr. Black took approval of the project to the trustees in May, a quarter early, prior to the planned completion of the test period of six months. With the trustees approval, additional capital became available to add a second VAX computer, creating a cluster to host the database in Oracle, and we started to distribute our users over both computers. I recall keeping graphic meters running constantly on my desktop to see how the system was performing.

Once the success of the pilot was certain, and with the approval of the trustees, my physician partner and I started to plan the official rollout for the system. It was a complex plan, beginning with getting the physicians in a physical area of the Davis Building to agree to transition from handwritten notes in the medical record to the process of dictation and transcription. The greatest utility gained through the automation was getting the clinical notes captured as discrete data rather than the image format. The image data was in the form of binary large objects (BLOBs), which means that an image was stored as a sequence of 1s and 0s and could not easily be sorted or manipulated by computer languages.

Our mantra at the time was "Capture as much of the patient encounter as discrete data to realize the greatest utility of the information." With discrete data, a computer could scan a patient record to look for clinical findings, which might trigger a notice of a critical situation, or remind the physician to check for a drug-drug interaction that might not be in the best interest of the patient.

An obvious next step was to launch the ACP workstations in each of the clinical areas where the physicians in the pilot program had their practices.

For example, the neurosurgeons were in the pilot group, so placing the ACP workstations in the Neurodiagnostic and Surgery areas was the first priority. In St. Luke's Hospital, the Clinic had what was termed the "Hospital History Desk." This unit was staffed around the clock to keep track of the Mayo Clinic history when a patient from the Clinic was admitted to the Hospital.

5 South	1
4 East, 4 South	2
5 East	1
OR Dictation Rooms	2
Medical Records	1
Preoperative	1
4 North	1
Postop Recovery	1
CCU (2 East)	1
PCU (3 East)	1
3 West	1
3 North	1
SICU	1
2 West	1
2 North	1
5 West	1
Radiology	1
GI Procedures	1
Mayo History Desk	1
3 South	1
Pathology	1
Surgical Records/Pricers	1
Cardiac Lab	1
Training Area	4
Operating Rooms	16
Emergency Department	1
Total	46

St. Luke's Hospital had its own medical record, so the Clinic history turned up in trash bins, laundry hampers, or just about anywhere. St. Luke's history stretched back to the early days of Jacksonville; it was founded by a group of women who felt it important for the city to have a hospital. The name St. Luke's was chosen by the founders, not as a reflection of a religious affiliation but because St. Luke in the Bible was the physician member of the Apostles. Mayo Foundation made the affiliation in 1987, but the Hospital had an open medical staff.

Prior to this, all of the other Mayo Foundation hospitals were closed staff, meaning only Mayo Clinic physicians practiced in them. There were a number of challenges to operating an open staff hospital with both community-based and Mayo Clinic physicians.

By putting a number of workstations at strategic locations in the hospital, we hoped to eliminate the need to circulate the paper-based Mayo Clinic record there. It would result in many economies for the outpatient practice and would reduce or eliminate the risk of losing a clinic record permanently when it was sent to the hospital.

A document from June 6, 1994, contained the initial rollout of workstations at St. Luke's Hospital to serve the needs of the Mayo Clinic physicians, planned to follow in the specialty areas of rollout at Mayo Clinic Jacksonville. The network wiring and the wiring closets with emergency electrical power supplied by the generators had to be built or installed before the workstations could be set up in the many locations. It is noteworthy that this plan was dated six months after the pilot began, so it was dependent on the outcome of the program, labeled "draft," and contained the word tentative in the heading.

As the pilot proceeded, more and more physicians embraced the technology, and at peak times, typically midmorning and midafternoon, we started to get calls and complaints about response time. One particular Monday in July, we had an especially frustrating day. The campus had grown and the support space in the Davis Building had reached the limit for telecommunications.

The Stabile South Building was originally built as a warehouse and powerplant for the campus. Some offices were built at the front of the space, facing the Davis Building, to house the administrative functions for Campus Planning and Projects. To accommodate the needs of telecommunications, space was designated on the second floor to house the new point of presence (PoP) and telephone switch that served the expanded campus. About the same time that the new telecommunications area was built, a new power plant was constructed west of the building. When the chillers were taken out of service, some of the connecting power lines were abandoned underground on the south side of the building and quickly forgotten.

When we received our second VAX to support the Automated Clinical Practice, we started our move towards high availability and located it in a portion of the telecommunication space. In installing the new computer, the technician failed to recognize the console was connected to a standard wall outlet rather than one protected by the surge protector and uninterruptable power supply.

For no particular reason, the forgotten buried power line insulation reached a point of breakdown and arced to the conduit, producing a power outage and surge that flashed through the entire building a little after 9:00 a.m. It also damaged the console terminal for the new VAX. The damaged part and the computer cluster worked fine, but after approximately forty-five minutes, one of the components would heat up, and then a thermal cutoff would occur. That second VAX would take itself out of the cluster, so all of the database and users were back to operating on the one, original VAX, which resulted in a huge response time slowdown. After the part cooled, it would begin to operate again. The second VAX would rejoin the cluster, and everything would begin to gradually increase to normal speed…until that part heated up again. And then the cycle repeated.

We did an "all hands on deck" call to the technical team, and everyone started looking for answers about why the performance had changed so dramatically. Near noon, the problem was discovered, and the console terminal was disconnected from the VAX, and the system resumed normal processing. This is but one example of the growing pains we experienced during the rollout of the ACP. When all was complete, we ended up on a platform that consisted of four VAXs and a daunting amount of disk arrays for storage of the clinical information.

Our bumpy experience made several things clear: Murphy's Law is true—if anything can go wrong, it will. His correlaries are true as well. It will go wrong at the worst possible moment, and usually cause the greatest degree of harm. Another rule of thumb: The more difficult a problem is to find, the simpler the problem. In this case, the computer had been plugged into the wrong power outlet. It was a regular outlet, not on the filtered power supply. When the surge of electricity hit, the damage was done to the terminal, thus creating the bigger problem.

Each of those disruptions due to electrical or mechanical problems caused us to reflect on our decision to automate the clinical process. Rather than be discouraged, we refocused our efforts on improving reliability. In an early morning staff meeting led by Dr. Black, one of our physicians said, "No one wants to go back to the paper chart. We want to help improve the reliability of the computer-based system!"

The work that remained was to implement the system to the entire outpatient practice, while improving the uptime and reliability of the system. We needed to grow the computer platform to support the growth of the practice, fine-tune the operation of the application for each of the specialty groups for increased efficiency, and come up with a means to cover the practice for downtimes, whether they were scheduled or not. How would we address these challenges?

CHAPTER SIXTEEN

The Rollout

We are becoming the servants in thought, as in action,
of the machine we have created to serve us.

—John Kenneth Galbraith

At Mayo Clinic Jacksonville, we developed a plan to roll out the ACP in the eight-story Davis Building, which housed the outpatient practice. The drawing on the right shows a schematic of the building (by floors). The areas in white still used the paper-based record, and the areas in gray had completed the ACP and no longer required the circulation of the paper record. Those areas colored gray crosshatch reflected the next priorities for implementation. This graphic was displayed periodically to administration and staff for updates on the progress.

ACP Rollout Priorities

Floor			
8th	Hem/Onc Endocrine	Neurology	
7th	Thor, Infec, Allergy, Rhuem	Cardiovascular	
6th	Gastro	Hyp/Neph N.S., GIM	
5th	Central Appointment Office, Scheduling Services Support Floor		
4th	Derm Ortho	PM&R CV/Th Surg	Psych, Sleep Neuro Diag
3rd	Urology Gynecology	ORL, Ophth, Gen Surg, Colorectal Surg	Exec, Internatl Plastics
2nd	Radiology		
1st	Registration, Administration, Medical Records, Xray Archives, Support Floor		

Legend
Paper
ACP Next
Complete

There were several steps in what became a standard process for implementing the ACP to the various specialties and subspecialties in the practice. We required the department or division to make a collective decision that they were willing to make the transition. From a practice perspective, all of the members of the division needed to be ready to move to dictated and transcribed clinical notes.

Operationally, the secretarial work model had to be reworked in order to identify those who were willing and able to become transcriptionists. Not every secretary was interested in, or willing to, transition to this new role; however, we were able to identify a sufficient number in each division so we could cover the resulting change in workload. In the facility plan, we identified space for the new transcription area for the division. Transitioning all of the physicians to dictating and transcribing notes required time, too.

Oftentimes a busy physician would dictate his notes between seeing patients, or he would see patients all morning and then dictate all of his notes at lunchtime. The problem with the latter approach was the delay it created because of the first in-first out queueing at the transcription service. Instead of a transcriptionist being able to keep the work flowing, completing clinical notes for the physician as visits were completed, there would be no work and then a backlog.

This approach created a delay for the patient; if the clinician at the next appointment needed the clinical information from the previous visit, it might still be in line for transcription. When informed of the trend, my physician partner made it a point to meet with the physicians and help them understand the delay they were creating.

Another issue was having the transcriptionists physically close to the clinical workspace. Being located at the end of the corridor closest to the physician's desk enabled interaction between the physician and the transcriptionist. To be most productive, it was important for the transcriptionist to concentrate on listening to the recorded voice and transcribing the information. Interruptions, even for a few minutes, created huge delays because of the time it took to get back to the point of work prior to the interruption.

These interruptions may not seem like a big problem, but the transcriptionist would lose the context for the clinical note. When she returned to the partially transcribed note, the risk of errors increased, possibly attributing the note to the wrong physician, applying the note to the wrong patient, or associating with the wrong work type related to the appointment. If the note makes it into the chart with one of these errors, a medical records employee could spend hours trying to get the information into the correct chart. If incorrect medical information was attributed to the wrong patient, the next clinician seeing the patient could make an erroneous diagnosis or prescribe an inappropriate medication or treatment.

Another challenge arose when physicians failed to sign off on an electronic medical record session. They might be paged away, or called away by a colleague, and then walk out while still logged into the patient's record. It didn't occur to them that anyone walking in before the session timed out could view or tamper with the patient record, with all of the privileges of the attending physician. If the session was still active, anyone could look up another patient's record with impunity, thus introducing a huge risk to patient privacy and confidentiality.

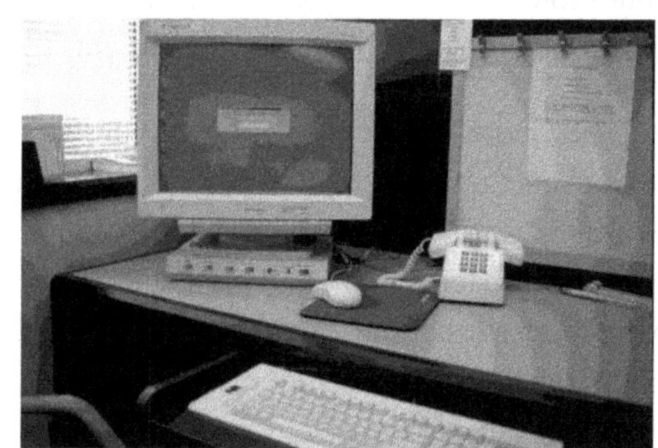
Typical installation of the physician workstation on an exam room desk.

On the technical side, open sessions created digital capacity problems. We had to find the inactive sessions and assume they had been abandoned. After so many minutes of inactivity, the technical team developed processes that would terminate the abandoned sessions, thereby freeing up memory and other computing resources.

Once a practice area had completely migrated to the automated clinical practice, the medical record was no longer routinely circulated to that area. The paper record could still be used, but we strongly discouraged this practice.

The process of converting all the physicians in an area from use of the handwritten paper based medical record to the computer based record with dictation and transcription, was preceded with pulling network wiring, installing workstations in the physician offices, then the exam rooms. In preparation for converting an area, we built the automation to enhance physician productivity as well as to include order sets for diagnoses, clinical notes, and charging for the visit.

For example, when a patient presented with symptoms for a urinary tract infection, there could be one or more tests to confirm the diagnosis. Once confirmed, a pharmaceutical formulary needed to be available as a reference, with alternatives for the physician to prescribe for the patient. And background checks were needed for any condition contraindications, drug-allergy, or drug-drug interactions that could cause problems for the patient.

The Cerner application suite was programmed to perform these background checks and to warn the physician of any potential problems. The applications were table driven but needed a perceptive computer systems person to build and verify the system performance. Mr. Charles Pugh did an outstanding job in collaborating with my physician partner and other division chairs to build the order sets and reference tables in the Cerner system during the rollout phase, and he continued to work patiently with physicians on fine-tuning the screens for their specialty practices many years beyond.

We completed the rollout to all of the outpatient practice by the end of January 1996. The nagging question after years of planning, work, and major capital expenditures was whether automation would affect the operational, clinical, and financial performance for Mayo Clinic Jacksonville. If so, what would the impact be? The answer would come in time, but we needed some experience with the paperless practice before we could ascertain the results.

CHAPTER SEVENTEEN

Biometrics

It's supposed to be automatic, but actually you have to push this button.

—John K. H. Brunner

The emerging issue of computer sessions with a patient's medical record being left open by a physician called away or simply moving on to her next patient was an unintended consequence of our success in getting physicians to use the computer-based patient record. While the physical security for Mayo Clinic was as good as, or exceeded, that of any corporate or healthcare organization in the country, it didn't address the concerns of computer security with a compendium of patient information left visible on an active computer terminal. Typically, once a patient was roomed, he stayed put until the appointment was completed.

Consider a patient in an exam room where the physician completed the prior patient exam and absentmindedly walked out to see the next patient. If the doctor did not log off the computer, the waiting patient had access to all of the electronic medical records that the physician could access. If the waiting patient wanted to "surf" other patient records on the computer, he or she could do so, and in the complete privacy of an exam room with the door closed. This potential gave a number of us many sleepless nights.

We began to formulate plans for addressing this issue. Locking or logging off a workstation was not difficult. But from the physician's point of view, it was just another time delay. Many doctors began to feel they spent a significant part of their time logging in and out of the system, adding tedious, nonproductive time to their already long day. We began to review technologies that would eliminate the problem. We considered using fingerprint biometrics, which emerged as one of the better understood and reliable methods available.

We also considered palm topography and face recognition, but both were prohibitively expensive for a single workstation. Whatever we chose needed to support nearly four hundred workstations in the outpatient setting. We aimed to keep the per unit cost reasonably low since we had to equip so many workstations. While it increased our capital costs, we had to avoid an accidental breach of confidentiality and possible litigation.

We settled on using a separate screen saver on each desktop, which would have a network tie to the Cerner user ID and password. When a physician approached a workstation in an exam room, or an area of the clinic that was exposed to the general public, he would place a finger on the fingerprint reader. Once situated properly, he would hit the enter key, which in turn captured an image of the fingerprint.

An algorithm would find the minutia points, swirls, and bifurcations and calculate a unique number. That number would be compared with the unique number generated by the image of the same fingerprint stored on the networked system database. With the correct comparison score, the system would verify the identity of the user, log him into the system, and open the screen saver, granting access to the user.

At the end of a session, the clinical user only had to hit a single keystroke (F9) to activate the screen saver, protecting the confidential information of the patient. Additionally, an automatic timeout would activate the screen saver, locking further access to unauthorized users. A physician or nurse could now access to the ACP through the Privacy Curtain system in one of three ways: (1) use a fingerprint scan alone, which acted as the user ID and password, (2) type in the user ID and use the fingerprint as a password, or (3) type in both the user ID and password.

Since the screensaver would be on every clinical workstation exposed to the public, we had to provide an alternative means to access the records in the event of the fingerprint system being down, and that was provided by option three.

Dr. John J. Mentel was the physician champion working with the project team in the development of the product. His feedback proved invaluable as successive waves of products and versions were tested. About the time he was engaged in testing these new products, he became the chair of the Foundation-wide Information Security Committee, and he served in that capacity for several years.

Each participant using the Privacy Curtain had to register two fingers, preferably one on each hand. When a finger was registered to a user, the information security officer had a process to ensure the clearest possible fingerprint image was recorded for the database.

The workstation at the right shows the workstation with the biometric reader in the keyboard. The registered fingers would be used by the computer algorithm to open the Privacy Curtain screensaver. The registration of two fingers was a precaution, in case one finger was unusable for a period of time, such as from a cut or burn.

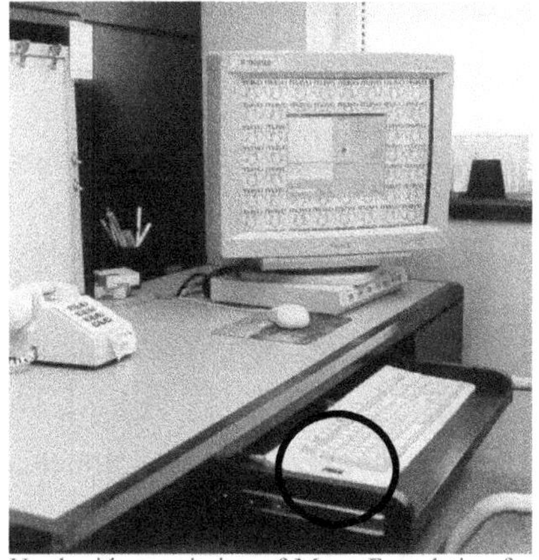

Used with permission of Mayo Foundation for Medical Education and Research, all rights reserved.

Once the system was production ready, we installed it in every physician workroom, corridor, and exam room. At one point Mayo Clinic Jacksonville was considered the single largest commercial installation of fingerprint biometric security in the world, both in the number of fingerprint sensors installed and the number of authentications per day. At St. Luke's Hospital, it was installed on every beside workstation, physician dictation area, and nurse workstation. With the installed base at St. Luke's Hospital, there were approximately eight hundred workstations secured with fingerprint biometrics across both campuses.

The features of the final product included security that covered patient information with a single keystroke and that saved the record in context, so when the physician returned to the EMR, she would start where she left off. For example, if the physician secured the record in the exam room after an appointment, returned to her office, and then accessed the EMR in the dictation area, it would open to the same place, on the same patient, and she could continue her work on the patient record.

It also allowed multiple physicians to share the same workstation, all the time maintaining the same context for each user. Once a physician used a workstation, the database data was cached locally to speed up the log-on process. The other active sessions on a shared workstation would be hidden from the current user, so there was no confusion about which record was active.

Computer technology in a medical practice brings some harsh technical realities from an active participating physician perspective. It takes a relatively long time to log on or log off a client workstation in dynamic medical practice. The high cost of physical space necessitates that multiple care providers share the same workstation, and logging on or off between clinical users on the same workstation is time-consuming, especially when a person is waiting to use the computer.

I participated in an Information Technology Fair at Mayo Clinic in Rochester in August 1998. The photo here shows me demonstrating fingerprint biometrics for the former First Lady, Barbara Bush in Philips Hall when she was a public trustee for Mayo Foundation. The

Privacy Curtain application was on the enterprise-wide network from the application servers at Mayo Clinic Jacksonville.

There are limitations to fingerprint biometrics that must be mentioned. There is a small percentage of persons who have very thin or fragile skin, where getting a clear fingerprint is difficult or impossible. Other individuals work in physical professions where the skin is exposed to chemicals or solvents, which also creates problems. Finally, producing a fingerprint is an outcome of the natural oils and the exfoliation process of the skin. In medicine, washing the hands between patients removes those natural oils and makes it difficult for the fingerprint sensor to get an image. The keyboard in every exam room had a small plastic case nearby with a sterile compound, so a clinician with clean hands would be able to touch his finger to the product and get a clear fingerprint image on the sensor.

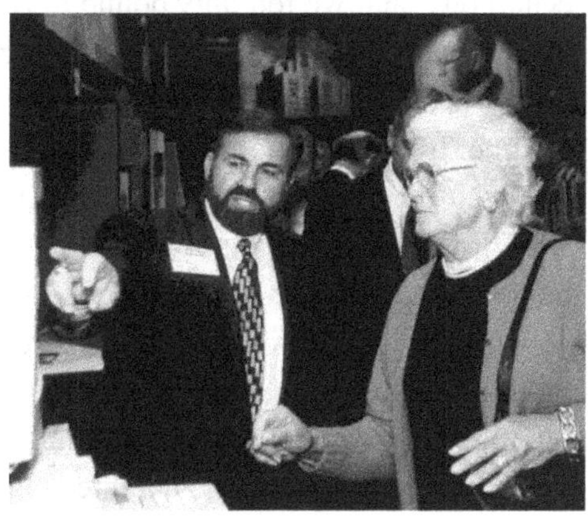

The author demonstrating for former First Lady Barbara Bush.

Used with permission of Mayo Foundation for Medical Education and Research, all rights reserved.

Even though the technology worked well in accomplishing our objectives, a couple of incidents caused alarm, bringing the use of fingerprint biometrics to a quick stop. The first incident happened without warning when Physician A placed her finger on the sensor, and the image was captured. The Privacy Curtain responded by logging her in as Physician C. In security technical jargon, this is referred to as a false positive accept. The application took the fingerprint and provided access to the wrong physician. Additional work ensued to improve the accuracy of the algorithm with tighter scoring criteria. The tighter criteria improved the accuracy and the application continued to work.

When you are responsible for all of information technology on a campus, this kind of occurrence plants doubts about the efficacy of the technology, and we felt duty bound to find a better means of accomplishing our objectives. A new technology that worked on the human biometric of the iris was being developed in the United Kingdom at the time. Iris recognition is often confused with retina scanning, the high-tech security measure often seen in James Bond movies and spy films. It is noteworthy that a limitation of the fingerprint biometric is the number of minutia points produced compared with that of iris recognition. Fingerprint technology at the time used 15-20 minutia points compared with 200-400 minutia points used in iris scanning. Ten times more minutia points is a substantial improvement in the corresponding accuracy to guarantee uniqueness of the identification of the user.

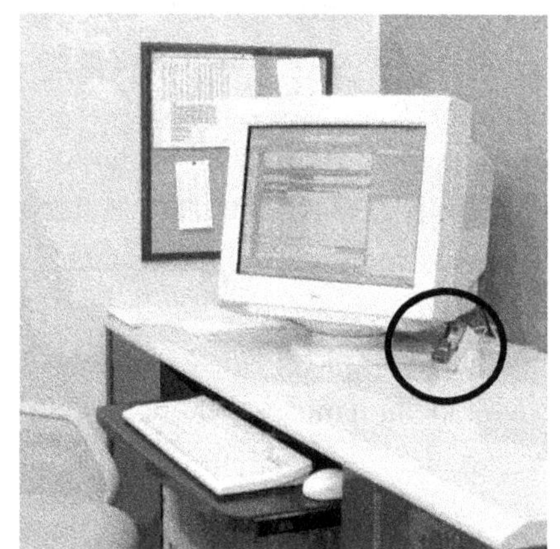

Used with permission of Mayo Foundation for Medical Education and Research, all rights reserved.

A workstation with Privacy Curtain and the iris scanner installed in an exam room in the Davis Building is pictured on the right. In preliminary tests, acceptance of the iris scanning was positive by those who actually compared it with fingerprint biometrics

The event that caused the eventual failure of the fingerprint biometric system with Privacy Curtain was a technical problem in the algorithm. The original software developer placed a "time bomb" in the software. The time bomb had some code that would check the time and date when activated. It was set to go off based on a preset date. When the date arrived on the computer workstation clock, the software was programmed to stop working.

The intellectual property had passed through the hands of three different companies, and the likelihood of finding the source code was considered impossible because of the changes in ownership.

From that day on, everyone had to revert to using Privacy Curtain with his or her user ID and password. The investment in fingerprint readers became useless. We considered other software and algorithms, but the technology infrastructure was dated and the replacement cost prohibitive. The Privacy Curtain system became a campus-wide application for single sign on and eventually controlled all workstation access throughout the Mayo Clinic Jacksonville campus.

CHAPTER EIGHTEEN

Time for Accountability

It has become appallingly obvious that our technology has exceeded our humanity.

—Albert Einstein

The rollout to the entire outpatient practice was completed by the end of January 1996. Now it was time to assess the operational, clinical, and financial performance of Mayo Clinic Jacksonville post-automation. What was the overall impact?

In 1997, when all of the accounting for the calendar year 1996 was complete, the financial results revealed that operations were the most favorable since the opening of the practice in Florida. One of the first concerns when I started my work in Jacksonville was practice

Task	Paper	ACP
Secretary calls the medical record for correspondence	45–240 minutes	< 3 seconds
Physician calls for a chart on a patient	30–120 minutes	< 3 seconds
Find last year's prescription dose for a patient	30–120 minutes	< 30 seconds
Call the chart for a follow-up question by a patient	30–120 minutes	< 3 seconds
Primary care follow-up visit at the Davis Building	24 hours	Same day
Distance to transport the medical record	9.3 miles	0 miles
How many clinical charges were billed automatically	0	80 percent

Used with permission of Mayo Foundation for Medical Education and Research, all rights reserved.

efficiency. This table, created by Mr. Chihak, illustrates much of the improvement realized through the automation, comparing the delay experienced in getting the paper medical record with the automation of the clinical practice.

The other significant problem not reflected in this table was the issue of only one person having access to the medical record at one time. The ability to have the simultaneous access by multiple members of the team caring for the patient is a huge contribution to practice efficiency.

Dr. Black challenged the Division of Financial Analysis to review thoroughly the impact of automation, with the CFO, Mr. Bolling, leading the effort. Their report surfaced, with little or no input from the Information Technology staff. The division assessed every aspect of the operations to determine the results of automation and the reduction of full-time equivalent employees while the practice was growing.

In 1992, when the notion of the automation of the clinical practice was proposed, the ratio of allied health staff per physician was 6.4. For every physician seeing patients, there were 6.4 full-time equivalent staff supporting him or her. In 1994, with the pilot program launch, the ratio of allied health staff dropped to 6.2 per physician, and dropped each consecutive year until it reached 5.1 in 1998. That is a reduction of approximately 20 percent of the allied health staff needed to support the practice over the intervening time.

The capital invested was modest in the beginning, but the figure grew quickly with the addition of networking equipment, workstations, computers, data storage, and information services staff. Additionally, there were operational expenses associated with the licensing and maintenance of the software and equipment. We budgeted the maintenance fees and program upgrades to grow at approximately 3 percent per year. Workstations rolled out in the early part of the prototype, and the pilot needed to be upgraded. The information systems staff added additional members, budgeted at 3 percent for inflation and projected to grow at an annual rate of 4 percent.

The projected savings were based on estimates since it was difficult to arrive at actual numbers in some cases. For example, by closing the loop, accountability for charges for all visits should have approached 100 percent; however, not all charging for every clinical service was computerized during this time. In view of not having everything captured at the point of care, we could only estimate lost charges. The savings from lost charges were conservatively estimated as 1 percent of the net revenue at the time of the analysis. Since the physicians selected the diagnosis(es), rather than an allied health staff coder, we believed that likely improved the coding accuracy, which in turn drove billing. Two percent of the year's evaluation and management (E&M) coding revenue was estimated as additional savings, and finally, the improved physician productivity was estimated as 2 percent of the annual net revenue.

We based the measured savings on the number of full-time equivalents (FTEs) no longer needed to do the present work or the same type of work as the practice grew. During the conversion to ACP, the number of patients and physicians increased. The cost benefits for the reduced number of FTEs were saved wages plus benefits, with an annual growth factor of 3 percent inflation. With the elimination of paper forms, the print shop closed, knocking those costs out of the budget.

Finally, the freed space enabled the practice to better utilize the buildings. For example, space previously used for moving and storing medical records was eliminated and relocated to a logistics warehouse approximately a half mile from the Davis Building. I recall construction in the spring of 1998, when the former medical records space was demolished and replaced with a phlebotomy area and medical laboratory space to better serve the patients. I felt the full impact when they moved the paper medical records out of the building: The transition to an automated clinical practice was complete, and there would be no return to the paper record.

With all the measures and financial analysis complete, it became clear that the internal rate of return (ROI) was well above the hurdle rate annually. When measured savings and estimated savings were totaled, the ROI was even greater than estimated. The cumulative FTEs reduced through the automation totaled 193, at a time when the number of physicians on staff and new patients was growing. The analysis concluded that the automation increased the time physicians spent with patient and reduced the time they spent on clerical work.

Dr. Black surveyed the physicians in the practice to obtain feedback regarding their satisfaction with the automated clinical practice. Eighty-nine percent preferred the automated clinical practice, 10 percent preferred the paper record, and 1 percent expressed no preference. Seventy-six percent believed the ACP was more efficient. The expressed concerns centered on the quality of the transcription service, the delay associated with transcription, and the electronic ordering process. Least of their concerns was computer slowness and downtime.

Looking back on that time, the vision for the transformation of the practice had been achieved, and we had changed the basic culture of the practice. First was the transition from handwritten clinical notes in the paper-based medical record to the use of dictation and transcription for capturing the information, getting it turned around quickly and back on the electronic medical record.

The second major transformation was moving the practice from the use of the historical paper-based record, a nearly century-old practice, to images on a computer screen and the attendant loss of the ability to add notations with a pencil.

The results of the financial analysis and the survey of the medical staff made our team feel proud about what we had accomplished through the automation. It was all the result of teamwork.

CHAPTER NINETEEN

Applied Informatics and the Doomsday Record

The only way of discovering the limits of the possible is to venture a little way past them into the impossible.

—Arthur C. Clarke

The success of the automated clinical practice was exciting to the staff, administrative support staff, and to everyone working with IT. Dr. Black aggressively pursued other technology applications to serve the practice. Almost all physicians were quick to embrace new technology with demonstrated clinical effectiveness; however, technology touted to improve personal productivity was a much tougher proposition. The automation of the clinical practice had passed that hurdle; no one talked about going back to the paper medical record.

With the ACP complete, Dr. Black wanted to discuss my focus on the long-term vision of keeping the Mayo Clinic Jacksonville practice on the leading edge of technology. One morning he brought a cup of coffee into my office and asked me what I thought about creating a department of informatics.

I said it was a great idea but suggested we call it the Department of Applied Informatics. Informatics as a term was coined by the British to reflect the delivery of health care using computer technology. I pointed out there was a lot of innovative work on informatics throughout academia; however, once it was published in peer-reviewed publications, how much was carried through to practical application?

In a subsequent meeting of the Board of Governors in August 1998, they passed a resolution to create a new clinical department named Applied Informatics, with my physician partner as the chair, and myself as the vice chair. We would focus on finding new leading-edge technologies that could be practically applied at MCJ to increase clinical and operational efficiencies. It is important to note that neither of us was relieved of any of our prior responsibilities. We were challenged to build a vision for the future with innovative technologies and applications that would expand on the foundation of the ACP.

Since we made the decision to configure our production system for high availability, rather than fault tolerant, it would be go down at scheduled times for maintenance. The planned downtimes were scheduled for midnight on Tuesdays and Saturdays, and typically lasted approximately two hours.

Unscheduled downtimes can happen whenever, although the technical staff did everything possible to prevent it, or at least limit an outage as much as possible. Since the systems depended on electromechanical devices, they would fail at some point and could cause an outage. The question was not if, but when.

In the early days of the pilot, we held extensive discussions about what the practice could do when the system went down. One suggestion that kept coming up was to print a paper copy of the electronic medical record at night and then distribute it to each of the clinical desks prior to opening. It sounded like a reasonable proposal, if it could be done.

I asked a programmer to set up a system to test the theory in one area. A relatively small family practice group (five physicians) had opened a paperless practice in Jacksonville Beach, in a building that was designed to operate with only the ACP. The ACP was immediately popular with the physicians and patients. One of the patients was asked how she liked using a computer-based medical record. Their response was, "This is Mayo Clinic! I expect it to be high-tech!"

One of my senior programmers offered to build a program for the test at the Jacksonville Beach practice. It would extract all of the medical records for the scheduled patients for one day, and then print the charts for backup use in the event the computer went down and the EMR was not available. He had the program ready to execute within a couple of days, and we set it up to run during the night, after the practice had closed for the day.

We had our answer. It took the computer system eight hours to locate and extract the entire record for each patient scheduled for one day. It took another eleven hours to print all of the extracted records and used over six cases of paper. There were only five physicians in that practice, so it was clear that this scheme would never work for the Davis Building outpatient practice with hundreds of physicians and clinicians. If the computer didn't fail, it would all be for nothing, and we would kill whole forests for the paper to print a downtime record.

We had to find another solution for unscheduled computer downtime, especially if it occurred in the middle of a busy day. I referred to this scenario as "Doomsday," and the concept of a standby record became the Doomsday Medical Record. We were afraid. Finding a solution became a top priority for the new Department of Applied Informatics.

I met with one of the most senior and talented programmers, who had asked to work with the new department on software development, and we outlined the following strategy.

We planned to build a system using data extraction and display in order to build a non-Oracle database, which would contain all of the clinical notes displayed as text. I specified non-Oracle so that a virus or bug would not be replicated in the new database if one creeped into the Oracle clinical repository. We selected Microsoft SQL because it was a server-based, relational database and enabled the use of the Microsoft Internet toolset for creating a web-based Doomsday Record.

The preponderance of Internet access made the Internet Explorer user interface a familiar context for the backup record. The programmer and I worked closely, and over the course of two or three months, we had a prototype ready to test. Security of the new application was replicated and driven by a security table from the Cerner application suite to minimize maintenance. The Doomsday Record name stuck.

The biggest change in relation to our earlier attempts was that the program pulled all information on every patient scheduled in the repository. With this attempt, we faced a back file conversion to load the base system, but from then on, we only had to insert the notes that were added in a given day.

The extract system would scan the Cerner database to identify what had changed from the previous day. All of the new information was extracted and added to the downtime database, so the database on any given day reflected the clinical information available at midnight. The resulting record, while not perfect and up to the minute, was better than no record at all. Plus it used the existing network and server infrastructure without dependency on the Cerner software system.

This is how the new doomsday record worked. If the Cerner system went down, a physician would use Internet Explorer to select an icon on the desktop. The system would prompt him or her to enter the user ID and password. The resulting open session would look for either medical record number or patient name to produce a list of qualifying patients. The physician would select their patient from the list, producing a list a clinical note types in existence. By selecting the note, the clinical text would open on the screen, and the physician had access to all of the notes that existed for that patient as of the previous midnight.

When I demonstrated the new prototype for my physician partner, he told me the staff did not like the term doomsday record, so we renamed it "Contingency Clinical Notes" or CCN. A few people suggested that CCN could be confused with CNN (the cable news network), but that turned out to be a nonissue.

Once the prototype was built, we checked the power and sizing of the software and processing requirements and determined it would fit on a server the size of a large workstation. When the extract was complete, we used data replication software and distributed it to strategically placed servers operating on uninterruptible power supplies.

The strategically placed servers assumed a failure might make either power or the network unavailable. For example, servers were placed in practice space, not in the Davis Building, such as the St. Augustine or Jacksonville Beach practices. On several occasions the dedicated leased network lines were accidentally severed by a backhoe or experienced other failure, and with the Contingency Clinical Notes operating in the St. Augustine facility, the practice was able to operate successfully, providing time to get the lines spliced. CCN kept the practice operational on a number of occasions for a variety of reasons for more than a decade. The location of the servers was a security issue since they were distributed strategically at campus locations, and one or more had to be located outside of the data center. We had to assume the contingency clinical notes had to survive a fire in the data center as well.

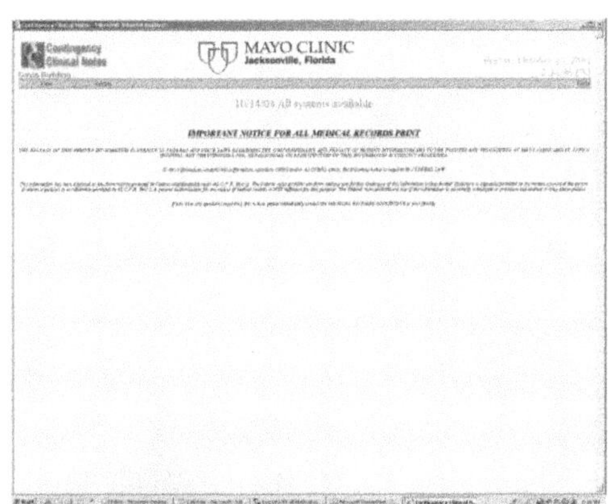

Initial Screen for Contingency Clinical Notes
Used with permission of Mayo Foundation for Medical Education and Research, all rights reserved.

At the heart of the issue was the single point of failure. As I worked with the programmer, we had to define the single point of failure from the vantage point of a physician with a patient in an exam room. If the physician attempted to access the patient record and was unsuccessful, then from his vantage point, the computer system was down. If the workstation was up and running, but the system was unavailable, then CCN could be used until we solved the problem.

Several years later, the Contingency Clinical Notes system was revised by the Applied Informatics staff to provide a downtime record, including laboratory, radiology, and nursing documentation as the hospital practice went paperless as well.

The entire clinical care team has embraced the paperless practice now. For example, a family member of the author was hospitalized last year. On the first day post-op, the automated clinical practice went down for an extended, unplanned outage. Nurses caring for the family member either didn't know or remember how nurse charting had been done on paper.

CHAPTER TWENTY

Referring Physician Office

Men are only so good as their technical developments allows them to be.

—George Orwell

From my first exposure to Mayo Clinic, I was impressed with the caring concern about preserving the practice. This was the practice of medicine established by William Worrall Mayo, father to William James Mayo and Charles Horace Mayo, and continues today, more than a century later. The practices established in Jacksonville, Florida, and in Arizona are extensions of the founding facility in Rochester, Minnesota. I feel it was commendable of the leaders to extend the corporate culture to the additional practices.

As the first, and perhaps the best-known, multispecialty integrated group practice in the United States, Mayo Clinic provides primary, referral, and tertiary care. A common misconception about the Clinic is that an outside physician, not a member of the Clinic staff, must refer a patient. In fact, approximately 80 percent of the patients seen at Mayo Clinic are self-referred, meaning they wake up with a medical problem and seek immediate consultation.

Here is a sample scenario. A person wakes up with a nonspecific pain in the abdomen, and she takes a couple of antacids. She feels better, but the pain doesn't go away completely. Over the next few weeks, the pain persists and begins to increase, but it's not debilitating. As time goes by, the pain grows more persistent and increasingly severe. She discusses the issue with her husband, who encourages her to see a physician.

She makes an appointment, and it turns out she is overdue for a physical, so the physician schedules the usual fasting labs and X-rays. The doctor performs the physical exam. All of the lab and X-ray results come back normal, and the physical findings are normal except for the abdominal pain. The primary physician decides the patient could have a gastrointestinal (GI) problem and refers her to a specialist. He writes a letter of referral and forwards the abdominal X-rays to the GI physician.

The gastroenterologist then performs a gastroscopy but finds no source for the problem. He suggests the pain could be related to the patient's heart since it originated in the high central part of the abdomen. Again, a letter of introduction and the results of the X-rays and GI exam are forwarded.

The cardiologist wants an electrocardiogram and treadmill test before he sees the patient. Six or seven weeks have now passed, the pain is worsening, and none of the physicians can isolate or identify the source of the problem.

At this point, the patient calls Mayo Clinic to schedule a thorough evaluation to find out what is going on. This can be a very frustrating experience. A patient with this kind of experience will end up as a self-referred patient at Mayo Clinic. The concept is that a Mayo Clinic Consultant is part of a greater medical team; consulting with colleagues about the patient often resulted in the discovery of a rare or complex problem, which they could solve by working together.

Managing patient referrals from outside physicians was a labor intensive, time consuming, and manual process at the time. With the Davis Building full of specialists, we were concerned with how technology might help with this referral process. By the late 1990s, the Internet was growing exponentially in commercial businesses, but development for health care providers hadn't really taken off.

We worked up the concept of building a technology platform that would serve the practice through the effective use of secure Internet technology tools. Amazon and other commercial and banking companies were using secure socket layer (SSL) encryption schemes to secure transactions between individual customers in their homes and businesses. Amazon was growing by leaps and bounds at the time.

The Applied Informatics team decided to build a referring physician program using the secure technology that would extend the referral base for Mayo Clinic Jacksonville to serve the primary service area. We focused on the 120-mile radius around Jacksonville, Florida. The decision on the distance was based on drive time and the ability of a patient to drive to the Clinic, be seen, and then return home without having to spend the night.

We wanted to encourage patients to come to Mayo Clinic from anywhere, but in cooperation with the other Mayo Clinic sites, we agreed to focus on the Caribbean Basin and the eastern portion of South America. Arizona was going to focus on Central America and the western portion of South America. Mayo Clinic in Rochester was considered a global draw.

The biggest concern from non-Mayo Clinic physicians was that if they referred a patient to Mayo Clinic, they might never see the patient again, thereby losing patients and the resulting economic loss. Referring physicians considered getting information back from Mayo Clinic a significant problem. Some harsh terms were sometimes used to describe that challenge, even though a summary letter to a referring physician was a part of the Mayo Clinic product and has been a long-standing part of the process.

The Internet application we envisioned would support a referring physician program built to select physician practices within that primary referral area (120-mile radius). We would target Mayo Clinic alumni since they knew the system and would have some affinity with the institution. The referring physician's office staff would be able to log into the designated website, provide the demographic information, and upload relevant documents regarding the referred patient from their office, along with preferred patient contact information and phone numbers.

The Central Appointment Office at Mayo Clinic would contact the patient to schedule the appointment and any related tests required to provide the Mayo Clinic consultant with the necessary information for their consultation. The Referring Physician Office (RPO) website would maintain a list of patients the physician had referred to Mayo Clinic, which enabled any of the clinical staff to check on the status of a patient in the process of being seen at Mayo.

When the results of the consult were complete, the original referring physician would receive a notification that information regarding her patient was available, which they could check on the portal. The referring physician could download the results and determine the next step for the patient. The key ingredient added by the RPO was building and maintaining the relationships between the Mayo Clinic consultants and the outside referring physicians.

The first version of the software application was available for testing about the same time people began to worry about a possible Y2K bug that was supposed to wreck all computer systems as the year 1999 dawned 2000. After these fears were squelched, we made our pitch to get administrative support for establishing an office with a supervisor and a representative. The representative would travel to meet with non-Mayo Clinic physicians in private practices to secure referral agreements, train office staff, etc.

The Department of Applied Informatics project description, dated September 2000, called for the development of a schema and application infrastructure to support a variety of services for persons or entities that have a relationship with Mayo Clinic in Jacksonville, Florida, as their healthcare provider or tertiary referral center through an *extranet.*

Extranet was a term that was in vogue at the time because it provided services much like an intranet internal to companies and organizations, but in this case it had a secure connection with an outside trusted entity. We planned to make it available on a variety of workstation types in various locations for non-Mayo physician practices. We aimed to establish an infrastructure utility to leverage the capabilities of the Internet and the electronic infrastructure established with the ACP to foster the development of a new business model for health care.

When we developed the plan, we designed it to fit within the Mayo Foundation presence on the Internet, and we built in support for use in Rochester, Minnesota, and Scottsdale, Arizona, if they chose to adapt a similar model.

It took time to hire administrative support, but once everything was in place, the RPO began to get calls from physician groups all over the state that wanted to join or affiliate. Word of the success reached colleagues in Arizona and Minnesota. At first the activities were coordinated, but before long the Referring Physician Office became an enterprise function that served all of Mayo Clinic locations. The software has since been reprogrammed, and it has become an extensive network application serving Mayo Clinic.

CHAPTER TWENTY-ONE

Capstone and Kiosks

Lo! Men have become the tools of their tools.

—Henry David Thoreau

At the annual meeting of the Healthcare Information Management Systems Society (HIMSS) in Atlanta, I met with Mr. Neal Patterson, chair and chief executive officer of Cerner Corporation, and I discussed our concept for the Referring Physician Office, using the secure Internet toolset. He said his developers were working on a similar concept under the code name Capstone. I expressed an interest in Mayo Clinic Jacksonville codeveloping the product with Cerner and then collaborating on the alpha testing for the concept.

By using the Referring Physician Application to create a new Internet-based business model, we built a core platform of features that could be used in a number of web-based applications to serve other clinical areas for our patients. Building a broader referral base for the relatively large multispecialty offerings in patient care was critical to our future operational and financial success. Once success in this important area was on sound footing, the next logical extension was to broaden the application base for patient services.

We defined our objective to develop an Internet-based application infrastructure to support a variety of services for persons or referring physicians who had a relationship with Mayo Clinic and/or St. Luke's

Hospital in Jacksonville, Florida, as their healthcare provider or tertiary referral center. We conceptualized a suite of secure services that would function on a variety of platforms, depending on the setting of the service.

For example, a patient who wanted to update his preferred address for correspondence had to be physically present with a registration clerk to make a change of address. It seemed logical for the patient to input the same information directly, rather than relying on a clerk, regardless of the setting. It would be important to verify the address as valid with the U.S. Postal Service, but that verification was easy to obtain. Patients could update or change the address from several settings if the application was available on the Internet. The change could be completed at registration, or at a kiosk in the Mayo Clinic lobby, or from a home computer, if the Clinic had established a relationship with the patient. We wanted to use the same application for any of these settings if possible, so we set out to accomplish that goal.

As we began to plan all of the applications that would benefit our patients and had the potential to work in a variety of settings, we quickly filled up a flow chart diagram that needed a tabloid-size sheet of paper to contain even brief keyword descriptors. For example, the section on payments grew to: view my bill, pay my bill, with debit or credit cards.

Registration information could be updated or changed, with opportunities to add more than one address if the patient desired. Insurance could be validated and updated if the patient switched providers.

Patient identification was another item we tried to make more efficient. Our application allowed a patient to use a magnetic striped identification card, which the Clinic would produce and send to the patient. The swipe card would enable a patient to walk up to a kiosk, pull up her appointment schedule, and print a new copy. Lost or changed patient schedules were a constant problem, requiring staff to reprint a schedule if it was lost or if new appointments had been added. By enabling this feature, we would alleviate the burden on our desk staff. Also, a patient would be able to cancel an appointment if necessary.

The magnetic card would be useful to identify the patient quickly at the kiosk. We envisioned adding a kiosk to each clinical area that required a check-in for an appointment. After self check-in, the patient would wait for a desk staff member to escort him to an exam room.

Before choosing the magnetic striped card for patient identification, we had explored the use of memory cards extensively with a large European technology conglomerate. The cards we piloted came in three sizes, with two, four, or eight kilobytes of memory. The cards would have been issued on an individual patient basis. With the memory on the card, we could include the entire patient record, including demographics, insurance information, the most recent health history, and associated documents.

A patient would be able to walk up to a reception desk or kiosk, plug his card into a reader, enter his personal identification number (PIN), and check in for the appointment. The added benefit: when the patient went to a non-Mayo Clinic Jacksonville provider, all of his personal and medical information would be available to the new provider.

The problem we encountered was the level of value added by the technology. Within Mayo Clinic, all of the patient information was available to other areas of the Clinic as the patient moved from place to place via the network. No other healthcare facilities within the U.S. were equipped with the card readers. Except for checking in to appointments within our facility, the card was otherwise useless.

Smart cards with encryption chips are just now being implemented throughout the U.S. We were nearly twenty years ahead of our time in our work with smart cards; however, we did recognize benefits from the magnetic-striped cards in the area of patient identification.

Cerner Corporation selected the code-word Capstone because a capstone is placed on the top of a stone structure to keep weather, especially in cold climates, from seeping into the structure below, which could wash out or freeze between the lower level rocks, causing the structure to crumble. In terms of computer architecture, Capstone was intended to be the crowning achievement of the integrated architecture assembled with the Cerner application suite. It would link our automated clinical practice with our two most important constituents: our patients and our physicians.

We built the strategy in phases of increasing complexity. Phase 1 focused on building and validating a secure infrastructure. Phase 2 included building a two-way communication mechanism for non-Mayo referring physicians. The third phase involved building a two-way communication mechanism to support telemedicine initiatives and initial experiments with accepting information from patients one way. And the fourth phase concluded with two-way, real-time interaction with patients.

Our work to support telemedicine had several notable features. Mayo Clinic Jacksonville had contracts to provide medical care at several senior living facilities. We attempted to use telemedicine technology to cover those facilities by electronically linking to them. When the new primary care facility was built in the Cannaday Building on campus, we included a command center so a physician could complete routine patient checks without having to leave the Clinic campus. We realized the majority of complaints could be handled effectively by using telemedicine devices.

Part of our search for technology included visits with technology innovators. At one point we received the telemedicine package used on space shuttle flights to track health issues of the crew. I am sure a completely new generation of telemedicine devices is on the international space station orbiting the earth as this is being written.

The final phase of development was directed at full two-way communication, much like what is now available on patient portals.

We planned to include a unique feature that would enable the physician to monitor a patient's health condition with devices that would provide daily measures. Diseases of respiratory distress, congestive heart failure, diabetes, hypertension, and others could be monitored with daily collection and transmission of information back to a central healthcare monitoring facility.

For a modest monthly subscription fee, we could establish alarm limits with a notification service to summon assistance for senior citizens living alone. Dr. Black hired a major consulting firm to determine the feasibility of the business model and assess potential patient service pricing models with sensitivity analysis.

We planned to provide services both Mayo Clinic physicians and non-Mayo Clinic/St. Luke's Hospital physicians via Physician Portal Services. Portal functions would include order status, additions, changes, and authentication; chart review and authentication; updates on patient status, clinical findings, progress notes, and other features aimed at increasing physician effectiveness.

Staff could search for medical literature and publications with Mayo search and medical library services such as Medline. Finally, a physician could ask for anonymous patient satisfaction feedback via the service.

The patient portal strategy provided three groupings of services, with those available to all at no charge. A second tier of services provided a Mayo Clinic staff member to monitor the health status of a patient for a modest monthly fee. The third tier offered ongoing patient health monitoring for a chronic disease state at a higher monthly fee, with the goal of providing some telemedicine monitoring.

The use of this technology might obviate the need for the patient to come into the Clinic on a recurring basis for such things at Coumadin monitoring, congestive heart disease, diabetes, and diseases of chronic pulmonary distress.

Providing services to patients over the Internet created a dilemma in our planning, because a number of services benefitted both the practice and the patient, providing efficiencies to both. For example, if a patient had an appointment but couldn't keep it, the practice could allow the patient to cancel the appointment and then schedule another patient in that slot if there was sufficient lead time. A cancellation created an unproductive slot in the physician's day if another patient couldn't be scheduled during that time. We decided to offer all services that were mutually beneficial to the patient and the practice at no charge.

The following services met this guiding principle:

- **Appointment Requests & Cancellations**. This feature enabled a patient to request an appointment for a certain time and date. The practice would contact the patient to confirm.
- **Automated Appointment Check-in**. This feature would be available on kiosks or a patient mobile device if he or she were on the premises. It would not be available from an off-site location.
- **Billing Review and Payment**. This feature enabled Patients to review their bills and pay online by credit card.
- **Diagnosis/Problem** -Searchable diagnosis and specific disease management recommendations have been available on the Mayo Clinic site for a considerable time.
- **Disease-specific Education**. This feature provided tailored information unique to each patient based on his or her current active diagnosis list in the electronic medical record.
- **Health Risk Assessment**. This web-based tool enabled a patient to answer a questionnaire and receive feedback regarding corrective suggestions to improve his or her health status.
- **Mayo Clinic Online Store**. Patients could buy everything from medical equipment, books, and educational materials, to logo branded products of all sorts.
- **Information for Your Physician**. The patient could answer this questionnaire online, providing family and social history and the reason for the appointment prior to consultation.

- **Online Registration and Insurance Update**. This allowed the patient to preload as much information as possible for the Registration and Billing Office, in advance of the scheduled appointment.
- **Patient Satisfaction**. This capability would automate the process of having the patient complete satisfaction questionnaires regarding the facility and the physician.
- **Prescription Refills**. With the automated clinical practice, an active medications list was available for patients to order refills and renewals of their prescriptions.
- **Schedule Review and Printing**. This feature enabled the patient to access and print his or her appointment schedule from home or from kiosks on the Clinic campus.
- **Sick Patient Symptoms**. Capturing the symptoms of a patient requesting an appointment was useful in determining the urgency of the request for the appointment. For example, the patient may need to see a physician in primary care practice, which is much less expensive than a visit to the Emergency Room.

We also identified services that would require Mayo Clinic resources (time, materials, and expenses) to benefit the patient. We were happy to provide them to our patients, if they were willing to cover the associated costs. What follows was our initial list of fee-based, elective services that we thought would be beneficial to the patient:

- **Annual Health Record on a CD/DVD**. A patient could receive a copy of his or her electronic medical record on a CD/DVD. It would be readable on any laptop equipped with Internet browser capability.
- **E-mail to His or Her Physician**. The time it takes for a physician to respond to email from patients puts it low on their list of things they like to do. Many physicians offered the option of emailing with patients declined.
- **Personalized Health Record Pages**. These pages were pulled together automatically at the request of the patient. They in-

cluded the patient's active problem list and were useful in helping the person manage his own health status.

- **Personalized Patient Health Book**. This personalized patient book would include sections relevant to her problem list with greater detail than the personalized health record pages. It would be tailored to the specific patient at that point in time.
- **Self-booking for Appointment Slots**. This feature would allow a patient to look at the appointment slots for a given physician, by date and time, and then book the appointment online.
- **Transplant Patient Monitoring**. The transplant program requires a lot of monitoring of patients waiting for a transplant, or of a patient who has received a transplant. This feature would allow members of the transplant team to check on a patient with near real-time monitoring devices.
- **Wellness and Fitness**. We envisioned a feature where patients could input personal exercise, diet, and food consumption, and then a Mayo Clinic staff member could make dietary and exercise recommendations based on current activities and diet.

We believed our plans for Capstone were elaborate and expansive. Many of the features are now available in the patient portal currently in use at Mayo Clinic, but some features still remain to be crafted.

CHAPTER TWENTY-TWO

The Medical Data Warehouse

The aim of medicine is to prevent disease and prolong life; the ideal of medicine is to eliminate the need of a physician.

—William James Mayo, M.D.

Dr. Black retired in August 1999, and Dr. Denis Cortese was appointed CEO and chair of the Board of Governors for Mayo Clinic Jacksonville. Change was in the air. My physician partner was invited to relocate to Arizona to take over leadership of their efforts towards going paperless and achieving the same kind of economies Jacksonville had realized with ACP.

Dr. Mentel was appointed chair of the Department of Applied Informatics, and he became my new physician partner as well. He and I both wanted to broaden the membership of the department, to encourage new and innovative strategies; whereas, my previous physician partner preferred a two-person department.

We worked out a policy for joint appointment, which was not new to Mayo Clinic. It essentially meant a person would continue to work in the same clinical area, with a portion of his time devoted to the Applied Informatics Department. We had twenty-two members; the majority were physicians from various specialties and sub-specialties, and the balance were administrative staff members, including Messrs. Keith Portell and James Houck of my immediate staff.

The Board of Governors charged the Department of Applied Informatics to leverage the wealth of data available in the clinical repository that had accumulated since the inception of the Automation of the Clinical Practice. We were to use the information to benefit patient care through the establishment and maintenance of a clinical research repository that reflected the data in the production system. The use of the repository was to support the research and education needs of the staff consistent with Mayo Clinic's vision and tradition.

We held the inaugural meeting in the evening, after the close of the clinical day. I discussed a research and development idea I had been kicking around in my head for several months. By this time, we had accumulated several terabytes of information in the ACP; however, there was no way for a physician to interrogate this clinical repository of information easily. Since the mission of the organization supports practice, research, and education, the consultants, as part of the faculty of the Mayo Clinic College of Medicine, were expected to conduct research and publish in peer-reviewed journals in order to achieve academic stature.

Conducting retrospective research on patient populations would be a relatively easy route to discover new clinical findings based on the records that had accumulated on our patients. A couple of highly skilled programmers might be able to craft a query about some aspect of a physician's practice, but it would be a one-of and not easily modified to look for answers to other questions. Dr. Mentel agreed we needed to develop a research tool for our physician staff members.

On the agenda that evening was my proposal to build a searchable database of all the clinical notes in the Cerner repository. The goal supported the Mayo Clinic mission for research with our consultants. A lively discussion followed, with most of the physicians agreeing there was no need for what I proposed. I expected my physician partner to support my proposal, but he kept silent. The proposal was almost unanimously voted down.

The department had been charged to do research and development, and so I felt I had some latitude to determine if what I was proposing was even possible. I was not convinced by the physician response and quietly went to work with Mr. Portell, my senior programmer, to see if we could create a solution. Like our work on Contingency Clinical Notes (CCN), we cloned all the clinical notes from the Cerner repository. The core infrastructure was established and working. The tricky part was building the needed indexes of information, the query tools, and a front end physicians could easily use. Keith built the front end using the Microsoft Internet toolset, which simplified training by capitalizing on the familiarity of other web browsing.

After several months of working on the development of the toolset and trial reports, Keith managed to build a working prototype. We had a lot of whiteboard discussions about how to extract and build the notes and statistical tables of the retrieved data on patients. We had to be compliant with the Institutional Research Board (IRB) requirements in managing the security for the system as well.

That spring we quietly showed Dr. Mentel what we had accomplished. We had built a test query database, and we tested the toolset for building an inquiry, searching for a simple, nonclinical term. The query resulted in a listing of patients with the occurrence in their clinical notes. Dr. Mentel was very excited. It was an "ah-ha!" moment, and he immediately saw the benefit of having a toolset that provided for free text searching of the clinical repository.

We spent the next several months building a complete conversion of the clinical repository for the medical data warehouse and refining the prototype toolset to make it production ready. We had to resolve a number of technical issues, like getting enough storage for the data and getting the applications in place to complete the nightly extraction and updates from the clinical repository.

By August we decided the application was ready to unveil at the monthly department meeting. Keith, as the developer and architect for the project, demonstrated the newly developed product to the assembled members of the department. We explained how to use the tool to interrogate the clinical repository to find the number of occurrences of a clinical finding, which would enable a researcher to determine if there were enough cases to warrant further investigation. It was impressive.

A consultant asked, "Is this the medical data warehouse that Reg presented at our first meeting back in January?"

"Yes," replied Dr. Mentel.

"This is awesome!" said another.

Keith demonstrated the statistical summary produced, comparing the statistical distribution of the query results with those of the total population meeting the search criteria. Default descriptive statistics by age, gender, state of residence, and more were tabulated and reported on screen and in a printable format. Consultants only had security clearance to look at clinical notes on patients in their care. To access clinical notes for a retrospective study, we needed to develop a protocol to be approved by the Institutional Research Board. However, once approved, virtually all of the chart review for the protocol could be completed on the computer.

That evening the group unanimously agreed to move the medical data warehouse into production, with a limited set of pilot consultants from the department as the first users. No one ever asked why we continued to work on the medical data warehouse after the proposal had been soundly defeated at the inaugural meeting.

About a month before year-end, the pharmacy received a recall notice about a batch of vaccines that were found to be ineffective. The pharmacist asked the Clinical Practice Committee what to do for the patients who had received the bad vaccines. The only way to identify those patients would be to perform a massive manual chart review of all active charts on patients seen during the previous few months. The manual effort of such a massive chart review was challenging to say the least.

Dr. Mentel, upon hearing about the problem, challenged Applied Informatics to see if the newly crafted medical data warehouse could provide some assistance. The numbers for the ineffective batches were loaded in the search tool, since they were documented in the clinical notes for each patient, and in a matter of minutes, we found 165 patients who had received the recalled vaccines. A list of relevant demographics was compiled, and all of the patients were contacted about the problem and offered revaccination if they chose. Administration and the consultant staff were very proud of what was now possible with the new medical data warehouse.

The following May the U.S. Food and Drug Administration recalled another medication. The medical data warehouse came to the rescue again. Mayo Clinic was able to contact the patients who were prescribed the medicine, advising them to dispose of the recalled product and to replace the prescription.

The labor associated with manual chart reviews to find this information would have been expensive, but when cast as a function of return on investment, the cost of developing and establishing the medical data warehouse paid for itself many times over.

These examples focused on clinical safety, which is of vital importance, but the longer-term implications on the retrospective research had even greater potential for benefitting patient care. With the basic search engine, everything from simple to complex searches could be tested using Boolean logic (a form of algebra) to build data samples from our existing clinical notes.

When the researcher saw the number of qualifying cases, she could then develop the protocol and submit it to the IRB for approval. Once the protocol was approved, the researcher and her team could begin the process of chart review for data collection. The toolset provided with the medical data warehouse was robust enough to support a number of simultaneous researchers, and it supported an unknown number of papers published in peer-reviewed publications.

On a parallel track, a group in Rochester was hard at work on a proposal to build an enterprise data warehouse to store all of the data captured by the information systems across Mayo Foundation. In a report to the public trustees regarding both of these activities, someone objected to the use of the term "warehouse" since it connoted a large, impersonal collection of patient information.

The person felt his clinical data was *entrusted* to Mayo Clinic for safekeeping. He recommended both collections incorporate a change of name from warehouse to trust. From that day on, the names of both efforts were changed. In our case, the medical data warehouse was renamed the Medical Data Trust and has kept that moniker since.

Our vision included more and more data and then the ability to do complex analytics with fuzzy logic engines. We imagined process analyses to discover new patterns of medical practice and economies by eliminating steps that seemed less productive in terms of clinical improvement. A laboratory for new analytics methods would challenge statisticians for years to work on techniques that may be unheard of today.

CHAPTER TWENTY-THREE

Blinded Data

The goal is to turn data into information, and information into insight.

—Carly Fiorina, Former CEO,
Hewlett-Packard Company

Dr. Black made it clear the Department of Applied Informatics was charged with keeping Mayo Clinic Jacksonville on the leading edge for technology, through research and development of new technologies applied to processes. Another task of our department was to foster relationships with local institutions of higher learning. In working with administration and the University of North Florida, we opened a part-time position for a graduate student in the College of Computing, Engineering, and Construction.

We were convinced it would be a win-win situation to have a student working on simultaneously on his degree requirements and the challenges of technology in health care. We hoped to bring the student on board in a full-time position after graduation.

We selected Mr. James P. Sweeney from the field of candidates. He attended classes on his schedule at the University, and spent twenty hours per week working on department tasks. His first assignment was with the Medical Data Trust (MDT). We asked him to create a new user interface, among many other enhancements that surfaced as physicians worked with the product.

Previously, the Health Insurance Portability and Accountability Act of 1996 (HIPAA) was enacted and signed into law. Entitled the Administrative Simplification act, Congress called for steps to improve the efficiency and effectiveness of the health care system by encouraging the development of a health information system through the establishment of standards and requirements for the electronic transmission of certain health information. In establishing the standards, the law gave patients the right to access their own medical information.

Additionally, the rule released in December 2000 stipulated the purpose of the regulations as having three major purposes. The first was to protect and enhance the rights of consumers by providing them access to their health information and controlling the inappropriate use of that information. The second was to improve the quality of health care in the U.S. by restoring trust in the health care system among consumers, health care professionals, and the multitude of organizations and individuals committed to the delivery of care. The third was to improve the efficiency and effectiveness of health care delivery by creating a national framework for health privacy protection that built on efforts by states, health systems, and individual organizations and individuals.

As part of this rule, standards were articulated regarding the de-identification of health information, which is useful for the analysis if the information is not individually identifiable. If we could strip all of our clinical notes of the protected information elements in our Medical Data Trust, we could share that information for clinical analysis or operational purposes with impunity.

I asked Mr. Sweeney to research how to hide or mask the identifiers from the clinical research repository, and he began to work on the problem. To accomplish our goal, we needed to identify and hide all occurrences of the following list of identifiers of the individual or of relatives, employers, or household members of the individual:

1. Names

2. All geographic subdivisions smaller than a state, including street address, city, county, precinct, zip code, and their equivalent geocodes, except for the initial three digits of a zip code if, according to the current publicly available data from the Bureau of the Census:

    a. The geographic unit formed by combining all zip codes with the same three initial digits contains more than twenty thousand people, and

    b. The initial three digits of a zip code for all such geographic units containing twenty thousand or fewer people is changed to 000.

3. All elements of dates (except year) for dates directly related to an individual, including birth date, admission date, discharge date, date of death; and all ages over eighty-nine and all elements of dates (including year) indicative of such age, except that such ages and elements may be aggregated into a single category of age ninety or older.
4. Telephone numbers
5. Fax numbers
6. Electronic mail addresses
7. Social security numbers
8. Medical record numbers
9. Health plan beneficiary numbers
10. Account numbers
11. Certificate/license numbers
12. Vehicle identifiers and serial numbers, including license plate numbers
13. Device identifiers and serial numbers
14. Web Universal Resource Locators (URLs)
15. Internet Protocol (IP) address numbers
16. Biometric identifiers, including finger and voiceprints
17. Full face photographic images and any comparable images
18. Any other unique identifying number, characteristic, or code

The covered entity does not have actual knowledge that the information could be used alone or in combination with other information to identify an individual who is a subject of the information.

The challenge of doing string searches for such identifiers as names, addresses, and phone numbers is a challenge but can be accomplished. The most significant challenge is finding all of the more common identifiers but then a reference to Mr. XYZ, vice president of General Motors in a clinical note is singular, and would nullify meeting the standard on all of the other identifiers. After several months of work and research, Mr. Sweeney was able to demonstrate a blinded database search.

Here is an example of how a blinded clinical note would appear with all of the HIPAA identifiers masked.

> MR. FIRSTNAME LASTNAME
> MEDICAL RECORD NUMBER
> DATE
>
> Mr. FIRSTNAME LASTNAME, a well-nourished XX-year-old male, presents today with chest pain and shortness of breath. He first experienced these symptoms recently while on vacation in CITY, STATE visiting his son FIRSTNAME LASTNAME.

Presumably the note would continue to discuss other presenting symptoms, family and social history, habits, medication list, diet, and exercise. Results of the physical exam would be detailed, with any abnormalities noted. Depending on the findings, consults with other specialists might have been ordered, and finally, the note would contain recommendations.

With this feature, researchers could review all clinical notes without the formality of having to develop a protocol, take it to the IRB for approval, and then begin the chart review process to find the relevant information for the question under review.

The process of creating a blinded database of the research repository was a lengthy process of the computer processing the entire database and blinding. Once the process of conversion was complete, there was a provision to audit the database to verify that every clinical note was blinded and did not have any personally identifiable information. We used sampling to arrive at what the law called a *safe harbor*, protection from liability.

Mr. Houck was the statistical expert in Applied Informatics for guiding our team through the complexities of the law regarding achieving a statistical safe harbor. He worked tirelessly on researching the legal framework and then building the statistical process for quantifying the outcome. He received his undergraduate degree in mathematics from Clemson University, and he had a master's degree from the University of North Florida. He was visionary in solving a number of problems through the years we worked together, and he always produced the highest quality work.

In order to scientifically prove the Medical Data Trust (MDT) data was blinded and met the safe harbor provision of the rule, a systematically selected random sample size of four hundred was drawn. This sample size was based on an estimate of the proportion of the population of notes in MDT that did not meet the definition of being blinded.

With no history regarding the actual variance of notes in MDT that did not meet the definition of being blinded, we selected the most conservative estimated variance. In addition, the error of estimation was set at 5 percent. A systematic random sample was chosen, since it was most appropriate for sampling a long list of notes (>10,000,000).

When the sample was drawn during in March 2004, four hundred notes were retrieved using the systematic (one in a thousand) process. We reviewed those notes to ensure they met the definition of blinded. There was one non-blinded element on each of two notes. (It turned out the non-blinded elements were typographical errors.)

This gives provided a note error rate of 2/400 or 0.005 or 0.5 percent. Given the sample size and the bound on the error of estimation, this result is statistically equivalent to zero. We met the Federal regulation for achieving a safe harbor by successfully removing the data elements listed in Section 164.514 and statistically proving "the probability of re-identification was very low."

Our safe harbor definition needed review and approval by some institutional committees and ultimately the Board of Governors. It was approved and our defined process became an institutional standard. All of the members of the Department of Applied Informatics were proud of the accomplishment of the blinded MDT. It served the institution well, spawning research questions by our clinical staff, with findings that had a positive impact on patient care, and it contributed to the academic promotion of our physicians.

Unbeknownst to the department leadership, Mayo Clinic had been nominated by an outside organization for the IT Florida 2005 Excellence in IT Leadership for the northeast region of the state award. Governor Jeb Bush presented the award in December 2005 in Orlando, Florida. The trophy was presented to the leadership of the Department of Applied Informatics: Dr. John Mentel, Chair, and Reg Smith, Vice Chair, and based upon the work of Keith Portell and James Sweeney.

IT Florida

2005

Excellence in

IT Leadership

Northeast

Mayo Clinic

Trophy Inscription

Despite the award-winning work in the department, the new CEO, who had replaced Dr. Denis Cortese, and another ophthalmologist took an action to the Board of Governors to close down the department that same month.

James authored a paper on the topic, which was published in the *Journal of the Healthcare Information Management Systems Society*.[2]

It was a bittersweet ending to the Department of Applied Informatics.

---

[2] James Sweeney, K. Portell, J. Houck, R. Smith, J. Mentel, "Patient Note Deidentification Using a Find-and-Replace Iterative Process" (*Journal of Healthcare Information Management*, 2005)

CHAPTER TWENTY-FOUR

Knowledge Management

True genius resides in the capacity for evaluation of uncertain hazardous, and conflicting information.

—Winston Churchill

Dr. Mentel dropped by my office one afternoon shortly after he was appointed chair for the Department of Applied Informatics. He challenged me with the following question: "As you peer into the future, what is the next big concept we need to be developing?"

"Knowledge management," I replied. He wanted me to elaborate. I went on to explain an industry trend to recognize that in a successful organization, the technologies involved in creating, disseminating, and utilizing knowledge create data that has asset value. This asset value is influencing how businesses are reorganizing to protect and secure the knowledge base that made them successful. That started a discussion of a concept we discussed for the next half hour, both of us chipping in ideas and concepts for further development.

In addition to the massive amount of clinical content in the data repositories, there is a body of knowledge around how Mayo Clinic Jacksonville operates and how it treats and manages patient care. Additionally, those repositories contain financial, patient, employee, operational, research, clinical, and process information. The many application suites and databases in the information technology portfolio operating on a variety of computing platforms and workstations built those assets.

In the course of operating, the amount of information being captured through automation is growing rapidly and adding value to that knowledge base at the rate of millions of transactions during the course of a day. Leveraging the knowledge being accumulated should increase the effectiveness and productivity in the clinical practice. The application suite could then be enhanced and disseminated to other practices. The resulting application code would create additional market value that could be used by other organizations to the greater good of more patients.

For example, the Cerner clinical application suite is the repository containing all of the clinical information on patients, and it has been accumulating information since 1994. That data contains details on all of the ordering, prescriptions, results, and clinical notes on patients, and it contains the observations and documentation by the various physicians involved in the care of any given patient.

That complex set of information also reflects process information, clinical outcomes, and financial activity. If Mayo Clinic and Cerner were to work in close collaboration on the information set represented in this example, the process could be refined with the clinical input from physicians and care providers. Cerner Corporation's engineers would need to refine the application.

The Knowledge Center was intended to be a physical space big enough to house these activities with practicing physicians, IT staff, and the informaticists and engineers from Cerner Corporation. Health care already had enough of what the accountants refer to as overhead, so we didn't want to fund the Knowledge Center from the practice or patient care billing.

A key concept was that the physicians would spend half or more of their time in patient care and dedicate the balance to refining the information about the practice, with a focus on increased practice efficiency. The algorithms would be engineered into the attendant application suite as a collaboration with the engineering team from Cerner.

We proposed that the Knowledge Center would be self-funding through the commercial products produced by our technology partners; after all, they would benefit from the joint development efforts aimed at making health care more efficient and effective, too. We felt patient safety and the quality of care would pay huge dividends through this focal point for all of the related activities.

Dr. Mentel and I collaborated on the Knowledge Center concept paper and built a business plan in what became a process for the rest of our time in the Department of Applied Informatics. The essential element in the proposal was to create the world's safest medical environment by leveraging the automated clinical practice at Mayo Clinic Jacksonville. We presented the concept paper at the Board of Governors meeting on August 9, 2001.

Dr. Cortese, who was CEO at the time, led the discussion of the strategic issues in regards to forming alliances with corporate sponsors, including the need for culture fit, and the different business motivators in for-profit versus nonprofit partners. The Board agreed the Department of Applied Informatics could begin to evaluate potential strategic information technology strategic partners and develop business options for consideration.

We engaged the Mayo Medical Ventures team to work with us on the development of a pilot project, with Cerner as the potential corporate sponsor. Cerner looked at our business model and assigned a physician from their company to work with Dr. Mentel and myself in refining a project for a pilot area to test our concept.

The result of those discussions resulted in a pilot for total knee arthroscopy. Dr. Mentel worked with the Orthopedic Department to identify a lead physician, and we collaborated on a proof of concept project. Mayo Clinic and Cerner Corporation entered into a Sponsored Collaborative Research Agreement to test the notion of building the first set of Executable Knowledge on the surgical procedure of Total Knee Arthroplasty (TKA).

If successful, there will likely be a second phase to broaden the resulting product to encompass all of Orthopedics. During the second phase, the development of a long-term business plan would be developed to establish the Knowledge Center as an ongoing integral part of the Jacksonville practice."

Cerner Corporation funded this proposed proof of concept with contributions "in kind" by Mayo Clinic staff engaged in the project. The project started in fall of 2003 with a contract-defined length of seven months. Cerner Corporation also contributed professional staff to Mayo Clinic for the collaboration effort that would engage the clinical staff in Orthopedics, Logistics, Administration, Nursing, Laboratory, Radiology, and other associated areas. A number of quality and safety criteria were established and used to quantify gains made through the process.

The performance measures included current state baseline and future state goals so improvements could be quantified. The project came to life under the code word Lighthouse, which became interchangeable with the term TKA (total knee arthroplasty) for the duration.

Quality and safety goals for TKA were set for such things as blood type and screen, post-op knee X-ray, blood type and cross match, bleeding time test, and transfusions. A plan was developed to automate the collection and reporting of a number of regulatory: indicators.

Goals were established as a measure of process improvement and a potential for the reduction to the cost of health care. Appropriate use of clinical resources for pre-op lab work, type and crossmatch, transfusions, and eliminating the need for a post-op X-ray reduced the cost of care.

Engaging case management to work on anticipating discharge planning was effective in reducing the length of stay. Having physical therapy work with a patient prior to surgery proved effective in speeding the recovery of the patient post-operatively. The process was successful beyond the imagination of many of the staff engaged in the project.

Flushed with exhilaration over the enthusiasm the project had generated, we moved on to the second phase of the project. All of the departments engaged in the project, especially Orthopedics, and we reported the outcomes and implications to improved practice efficiency, patient safety and quality, reduced expenses, and clinical outcomes to the Board of Governors. The summary was accepted with kudos; however, a change in leadership necessitated a hold on the next phase.

Dr. Denis Cortese was promoted to the position of president and chief executive officer for Mayo Clinic, and he relocated to Rochester, Minnesota. The search for his successor in Jacksonville was under way, and it would take several months to select the CEO. The Board thought it prudent to secure the new CEO before further work on the Knowledge Center proof of concept project continued.

Dr. Mentel went on to write extensively about the Knowledge Center concept, with the encouragement and blessing of the CIO and administrative leadership for IT.

I was invited to the enterprise role of Administrator of the Advanced Technology Innovation and Planning Office with staff assigned at the three major Mayo Clinic sites.

CHAPTER TWENTY-FIVE

Advanced Technology Innovation and Planning Office

You can use all the quantitative data you can get, but you still have to distrust it and use your own intelligence and judgment.

—Alvin Toffler

In 2005 Mayo Clinic set a corporate direction to draw the Florida and Arizona practices into a closer relationship with the founding site in Rochester, as a single enterprise with all three major sites operating as one Mayo Clinic. Information Technology was one of the first administrative areas to shift operating structure, becoming a shared services organization serving all sites.

An individual's work location did not necessitate relocation to one of the other campuses, though. For example, the administrator overseeing the data centers did not have to relocate to Minnesota even though there were more computing resources and data centers in that location.

The chief information officer invited me to the Rochester campus to discuss an idea he had for an expanded role for me in the new enterprise organization. He wanted me to serve as the Administrator of the Advanced Technology Innovation and Planning Office. My office would remain in Jacksonville, but I would involve travel to the other sites. I would have 2.5 full-time employees based in Jacksonville, with staff at the other sites, and I was promised that some portion of their time would be given over to the work of the office.

The staff from the other sites served in full-time leadership positions already. The promised relief for time to work on the advanced technology never materialized; nevertheless, we held an inaugural meeting in Jacksonville for all the members of the office in November 2005. We spent two days getting acquainted in face-to-face meetings and planning for anticipated activities.

One of the first needs to emerge in the following weeks was collaboration tools. Media services operated four full-time video conferencing facilities, with a video director at each site assisting with the technology. They were online from 6 a.m. until 7 p.m. EST, Monday through Friday, and still getting everyone together for a meeting between three sites was a problem. Getting time in these professionally equipped rooms was a challenge.

With the emergence of high-speed networking, we wanted to link up and collaborate from our office desktops. Over the next several months, we tested a half dozen products, with varying degrees of success. We wanted the ability to have ad hoc meetings with little notice. The group working on IT Education had already installed a production system, but it was limited to a maximum of four or five talking heads. The teachers would talk, and everyone else would observe.

We found and piloted a system for a year that allowed team members from disparate offices across the Foundation to meet virtually. It offered full document sharing, white boarding, visual displays, and even included a virtual backstage so speakers could message without those in attendance knowing. That project was called desktop collaboration, and we became highly skilled in use of the application package. Our demonstrations at the sites played a role in the Department of Research licensing the package and using it for the application of research education.

An ongoing problem that had dogged the practice since the early days of the automation in Jacksonville was the amount of time spent waiting for the computer to log on and log off. In Jacksonville we had tested fingerprint biometrics as a possible means to automate the process. We characterized our project as "Rapid Log on/Rapid Log off," and we envisioned using a unique token to track the presence of the physician.

For example, if we could "register" a unique identifier on a cell phone, we might be able to use a Bluetooth sensor on a workstation to know that Dr. XYZ was now in the exam room and ready to use the workstation. A screen would pop up, indicating Dr. XYZ was ready to use the computer. If he or she entered a personal identification number (PIN), the computer would open up to the current patient's chart. We would already know which patient was assigned to that room.

Sounds easy and straightforward doesn't it? However, here were some of the issues we faced. To access the unique identifier on a cell phone would also allow a hacker to "clone a phone," which is a Federal crime with heavy consequences. Bluetooth might enable it, but the early mobile phones with Bluetooth didn't always produce a "heartbeat" signal. So a physician might walk up to a workstation, but without the signal, the computer wouldn't open.

A couple of years before I retired, a number of physicians were questioned about their biggest complaints, and the leading problem cited was they spent too much time doing clerical/keyboard entry activities. This matter is perhaps one of the most chronic and irritating problems physicians face with automated systems today—too much keyboard entry and too many mouse clicks.

Another challenge the Office tackled involved the amount of computing resources sitting idle on desktops during and after the business day. The CIO and we believed a large quantity of computing cycles could be harvested and used for other computing needs. The technology is called grid computing.

The desktop would have a screen saver application to protect the user information whenever it wasn't in use. When the workstation was quiet, it would send a signal to another computer, which parcels out computing packages. These packages would be assigned to the idle desktop, which in turn would compute the task it was given and return the results to the assigning computer, and then signal it was free to do another task. The next task would be sent to the desktop for computation.

If you returned to your office and needed the computer, an interrupted task would be sent back incomplete to the controlling computer with the message, "I was unable to complete this task." The controlling computer would then send the same work to another idle computer.

By working at problem solving in grid computing, massive amounts of idle computer time could be harvested and applied to other constructive work. Bioinformatics and Medical Informatics research were two areas that could utilize this computing resource. Grid computing could be used as a cost effective source of processing power through the marshaling of unused computing resources.

Harnessed together, unused desktop workstations compute capacity can be used to process many types of computing intensive applications. These applications normally rely on high performance computing (HPC) resources, such as supercomputers, to process jobs, but with grid computing these jobs can be processed at supercomputer speed.

The majority of Mayo Clinic Jacksonville computers were being used during normal working hours. We estimated the computing resources were unused approximately 128 of the 168 hours available each week. A 1 GHz Pentium 4 workstation performed 1 billion floating-point operations per second. Floating-point operations involved fractional numbers; therefore, they took longer to compute than an integer operation. FLOPS (Floating-point Operations Per Second) were a common benchmark for rating the speed of microprocessors.

If only 50 percent of the four thousand workstation 1 GHz processors were used, the combined processing power would equal approximately four trillion numeric operations per second (4 Teraflops). If the utilization increased to 100 percent, that number would increase to 8 Teraflops. If we took the same utilization percentages of 50 percent and 100 percent and applied them to all workstations available in Mayo Clinic, the aggregate total processing power would reach between 144 and 288 Teraflops.

Given this potential for computing power, the Advanced Technology Innovation and Planning Office (ATIPO) piloted the technology. We found the grid would harvest unused CPU cycles on workstations throughout each Mayo campus and would provide a computational resource for the research community. We concluded the application of harvesting these idle computer cycles would address the need and better utilize these resources.

Our office also worked to establish a framework for an information technology enterprise architecture. We set goals for the framework: have a common look and feel for all patients, regardless of their location, deliver economies of scale, leverage assets, support mobility and collaboration for the consulting staff, and focus on effectiveness in the delivery of patient care. The work was seminal but established overarching principles to guide the information technology architecture. That work continues today under different leadership.

CHAPTER TWENTY-SIX

Socrates and Ask Mayo Expert

True wisdom comes to each of us when we realize how little we understand about life, ourselves, and the world around us.

—Socrates

I had not been the Administrator of the Advanced Technology Innovation and Planning Office for long when the CIO approached me to discuss an issue that had surfaced, referred to as a *code purple* event. Code purple was a term used for a result or diagnosis that could be semi-urgent and potentially serious or even life-threatening if the patient's care wasn't managed carefully.

An example would be idiopathic thrombocytopenia purpura. Idiopathic means no one knows why it occurs but the immune system starts identifying blood platelets as defective and the spleen responds by removing them from the blood. The normal range for the platelet count is 150 to 450 thousand platelets. A critically low platelet count can be an indicator of numerous other causes so getting an accurate diagnosis is vitally important. If left untreated there is a risk of a critical brain bleed or an internal bleed out. Once the condition is identified in a patient, it typically is added to his or her active diagnosis list and referred to as a code purple diagnosis.

"Reg, you know the technology. Is there something we can do with our technology platforms to raise our level of awareness on patients who may have an active code purple diagnosis?"

"I don't know, but let me spend some time thinking about our technology and platforms and see what I can come up with."

I blocked some time on my calendar to research some features of our technology and began to work on a draft plan based largely upon my knowledge of the Cerner application architecture in Jacksonville.

The schema I worked out went something like this: A relatively small number of patients are active at any given time, so the new system would build a list of active patients and use it as a work list. As results were produced by Departmental Clinical Systems, they would be sent to the clinical repository, typically through an interface. The data might be numeric or character in content; nevertheless, I postulated some kind of rule engine would examine the data to see if it met defined criteria for different kinds of conditions or diagnoses.

The active patient list would be used to review all clinical results on the patients. A rules-based engine would only need to see what had changed on the patient since the previous day. The results would be compared with the code purple condition database. If a match was found, a message would be generated and sent to an external tracking system. The outbound message would contain all the pertinent data regarding the patient, including the medical record number, ordering physician, code purple condition, and the source system.

The external tracking system would collect the messages and index and store them in a message database. If the physician had already been notified of his patient with the code purple condition, it would be stored as a sent message. Nobody likes to receive multiple notifications for the same item, especially if it has already been dealt with successfully. If the physician had not received a notification, then a code purple condition message would be sent.

In discussing this draft proposal with the CIO, he connected me with one of the top cardiologists in Rochester to discuss the enterprise learning system to see if my proposed plan could be linked. We talked about the two systems and immediately saw the benefit of coupling them, so we took on the challenge of bringing them together into a unified application.

When a physician receives a code purple notification message, a text arbiter would check the index of terms. The index would be a file of the code purple terms and the physicians within Mayo Clinic who had the most current expertise for the term. The physician involved in the care of the patient with the newly diagnosed code purple item would be offered a list of subject matter experts with contact by phone or pager, frequently asked questions and answers regarding the code purple diagnosis, clinical guidelines, self-assessments, publications, and other pertinent information.

We needed a name for this emerging system. I recalled the Greek philosopher Socrates's quote that the beginning of true wisdom was to know the limitations of one's knowledge. And so we settled on Socrates as the system name.

Since code purple conditions were rare in the general population, physicians didn't treat them frequently, and getting up to speed with the latest in research and management of the conditions would leverage the wealth of knowledge and expertise within the consultant staff. The Socrates portion of the enterprise learning system was characterized as "How Mayo knows what Mayo knows." Providing the physician with a variety of source information and materials was named "Ask Mayo Expert."

Once we developed the concept paper, the CIO shared it with administrative leadership, and the leading cardiologist and his administrator were working with me on building it into a business plan. The preliminary business plan hit a responsive chord with one of the benefactors, and the next thing we knew, a sizeable donation had been made to the development office specifically to underwrite the cost of developing Socrates.

We built the system to address the variance in EMR systems at each of the three major sites. Florida was on the Cerner architecture, Rochester was on the GE Centricity system, and Arizona was on a much older version of the GE Centricity system. We planned to convert the Arizona campus to the Cerner EMR. Rather than build the system for both EMRs, we planned to implement Socrates after the conversion to the Cerner system was completed.

The beauty of this system was that several tiers of educational services were available to each member of the consulting staff. For example, a consultant in Florida might find a notification in his clinical inbox regarding a current patient with a code purple condition. He might be comfortable managing the case himself; however, if he had not seen a patient with that condition in several years, he might like to discuss the case with another member of the consulting staff who had more experience with it.

The notification message would include a hyperlink to an expert on the condition if the physician wanted to discuss the case by phone. It would also link a physician to a panel of the leading experts in the consulting staff directory, which would contain all of their contact information.

Alternatively, the doctor might prefer to see the latest clinical information from the National Library of Medicine, or even take a short video course on managing the condition. In short, the system presented the physicians with a variety of options to become more current on rare or esoteric patient conditions.

The full list of options included, in the following order: immediate contact with a subject matter expert, frequently asked questions regarding the condition, clinical guidelines for the care and treatment of the patient, self-assessments, key things to know about the condition, and finally relevant publications in peer-reviewed medical journals.

We held a couple of daylong planning sessions in Rochester, with representatives of several divisions from Education and Information Technology present. Our plans included discussing connections to the global address list and the telecommunications system for presence detection. Presence detection was viewed as a critical piece of the technology because it would enable the ability of the enterprise learning systems to know presence by where a consultant most recently answered a telephone call or logged on to the network system.

One of the toughest questions to resolve was how to determine who had the expertise within the organization. We relied on individual clinical departments and divisions to build the the list of experts for a given set of problems.

For example, the Department of Cardiology determined which diagnoses needed to be listed as code purple conditions and which of the consultant staff at all three sites had the qualifying expertise to be listed as an expert for each given problem. If the highest ranked expert wasn't available, which consultant would be listed next?

Within a year the first of the code purple diagnoses were built and tested for reliability in detecting the conditions and properly completing the notification process as originally proposed. The Ask Mayo Expert system incorporating the Socrates code purple discovery mechanism and notification application continued as a production system at the time of my retirement.

The team involved in building this complex system included many of the staff from all of the campuses. The openness of the physicians, administrative staff, Information Technology staff, clinical staff, and others involved was remarkable. Once we clearly established the objective through the vision documents, everyone drawn into the project, from pilot to successful implementation of the first few code purple rules, worked together in a large-scaled collaboration for success. The names of all the staff engaged are too numerous to detail, but all can be proud of what we accomplished for the safety of our patients.

CHAPTER TWENTY-SEVEN

Care Connectivity Consortium

Share your knowledge. It is a way to achieve immortality.

—Dalai Lama XIV

The beginning of the Care Connectivity Consortium has an interesting origin. It grew out of an idea by the CIO at Mayo Clinic in 2007. He invited all of the leading technology companies to Rochester, Minnesota, with the goal of seeking a premier set of partners. During the course of the year, executives traveled to Minnesota to learn about the technology opportunities presented by collaborating with Mayo Clinic.

Intel, IBM, Cisco, Microsoft, Oracle, Avaya, GE, Hewlett-Packard, Dell, and Lucent Technologies made the trip. The typical program for these visits to Mayo Clinic included a greeting by the CEO and President. Information Technology Division chairs and their physician partners attended. Overviews with walking tours of the campus, luncheons, and dinners were included as opportunities for networking and discussion of possible future relationships.

The CIO liked the idea of convening a summit meeting of IT-related companies, with the IT and administrative leaders from Mayo Clinic in this case, to discuss the potential benefit of partnering with Mayo Clinic. To entice the representative executives to say yes to the invitation, he planned a summit at a resort in Phoenix in February.

It would be warm and sunny, with ample opportunities for golf, relaxation, and networking. It would be hard for executives to turn down this invitation.

The group convened in the Arizona resort and discussions ensued. After a couple of days talking about the direction of health care across the nation, and listening to a pitch about partnering with Mayo Clinic to develop new technologies for health care, the technology executives responded. They said the problems being addressed at Mayo Clinic were not unique. They requested that Mayo bring together the leading health care providers in order to develop a consensus about the leading problems with technological solutions.

Once those leading problems were identified, the companies would be willing to work together on building new and innovative technology solutions. With that response, the CIO faced a new challenge. How would he get the major players together, and how would they arrive at a consensus of where health care needed to go in the near and long-term future?

Mayo Clinic hosted another summit for three days in November 2008. The Clinic invited all of the major academic centers and large healthcare providers, in addition to technology companies. The first day and a half was devoted to discussions and work with the represented healthcare providers to arrive at a stated direction and consensus. Then the technology companies would arrive, with the hope that a partnership between both groups would emerge, with consensus about the leading problem(s) to be addressed as an outcome of the summit. The CIO felt it was a risky strategy on his part because he wasn't sure they would achieve a consensus about an agenda.

The outcome of this summit emerged as the Healthcare IT Standards and Interoperability Coalition with two major initiatives. The first focused on the need for a universal patient identifier, and the second addressed the exchange of medications, allergies, and problems across the healthcare ecosystem. This mixed group of IT companies and healthcare providers scheduled monthly conference calls to discuss these topics, develop position papers, and draft responses to notices of proposed rulemaking from the Office of the National Coordinator (ONC) for Health IT at Health and Human Services (HHS) and the Centers for Medicare and Medicaid Services (CMS).

Ironically I was leading a group with quite a different mission as Administrator of the Advanced Technology Innovation and Planning Office, an enterprise position, reporting directly to the CIO with staff at the three major Mayo Clinic campuses.

The launch of the Coalition in November 2008 coincided with the election of Barack Hussein Obama as the forty-fourth president of the United States. With control of Congress, the Health Care Information Technology for Economic and Clinical Health (HITECH) Act, as a part of the broader American Recovery and Reinvestment Act of 2009, was signed into law with the goal of stimulating the American economy, which was experiencing the worst recession since the Great Depression.

The focus of HITECH was to encourage the adoption of electronic medical records and the associated infrastructure to provide safer, high-value, coordinated care through the seamless interoperability of clinical information. Widespread adoption of electronic medical records was one of the goals for hospitals and medical practices. Funds were earmarked to incentivize physicians to help offset the capital required for the investment in the technology.

In February the president signed the Affordable Care Act into law, and the monthly conference calls for the Healthcare IT Standards and Interoperability Coalition began. The CIO asked me to assume the ongoing responsibility of keeping track of the agenda and attendance, and of circulating the correspondence electronically. It was a challenge since I wasn't a participant in any of the previous meetings in Arizona or Rochester.

For the first two years, we had interesting discussions and attendance was good. One of our first activities was to draft position papers in response to the Office of the National Coordinator for Health Information Technology.

In the fall of 2009, three groups volunteered to go in depth on some topics and produce position papers reflecting the recommendations of the Coalition. Our CIO tried to get them in front of the right audience, with marginal success.

In 2010 a second round of topic groups met for several months, outlining some of the key topics to research in greater depth, again producing position papers and recommendations.

In the fall of 2010, the Coalition decided to gather at one of the provider sites to reenergize the group and determine how they could gain more traction, get in front of a more powerful audience, and make a greater impact. The Coalition members, which included both health care providers and technology companies, planned to meet at Intermountain Healthcare in Salt Lake City for two to three days to collaborate and plan.

In the weeks after the New Year, I injured my back. By the time I was supposed to leave for the meeting, the pain had forced me into a wheelchair. On the last day of meetings, when I should have been in Salt Lake City with the Coalition, I was in the Emergency Department, where the doctors informed me that I needed emergency back surgery.

Following the Salt Lake City meeting, the CIO called and asked me to put together some thoughts about conducting a health information exchange between five of the Coalition provider members. He was going to fly to a meeting with the CEO of Kaiser Permanente and Intermountain Healthcare to discuss how we might collaborate on the exchange of patient identifiers and meds, allergies, and active problem lists.

I remember putting together the draft over a weekend and finishing it on Monday. I was scheduled for back surgery at 4 p.m. that Monday, so I went into work in the morning, completed the draft before noon, and sent it off. That afternoon I went on medical leave and did not return until late March.

When I returned, I was briefed about the development of a new group called the Care Connectivity Consortium. The seminal document I had submitted before my medical leave had grown into a collaboration between Kaiser Permanente (Oakland, CA), Geisinger Health System (Danville, PA), Group Health Cooperative (Seattle, WA), Intermountain Healthcare (Salt Lake City, UT), and Mayo Clinic.

The start of the organization was announced at the National Press Club in Washington, D.C., on April 6, 2011. The CIO asked me to be the project administrator representing Mayo Clinic, but having authored the core of the agreement, I was active in all of the workgroups for the Consortium.

There were some notable challenges for the members of these organizations in working together since they used disparate EMRs. Kaiser Permanente was the largest organization, using the EPIC electronic medical record, with eight instances of the EMR, one serving each of its regional corporations. Group Health Cooperative and Geisinger Health System both used EPIC, but Geisinger also operated the health information exchange for the state of Pennsylvania. Mayo Clinic used two EMR platforms, with GE Centricity servicing the Rochester campus and Cerner servicing the Florida and Arizona campuses.

The team at Intermountain hosted all the development efforts and engineered a very robust and well-architected system for the exchange of information between sites. Using an internal cross-indexed identifier, information could be exchanged between any of the Consortium members. For example, if I were traveling to southern California and was involved in an accident, and I showed up at a Kaiser Permanente hospital, the physician at Kaiser could request my medical record from Mayo Clinic if I had consented to the health information exchange.

She would have full access to all my information, active problem list, allergies, and medications and could treat my problem without having to repeat all of the studies already documented in my medical record. When I returned to my Mayo Clinic physician, I could tell him about the problem I had while traveling. The Mayo Clinic physician would be able to pull the information from my medical experience at Kaiser Permanente, pulling the Kaiser Permanente medical record into the Mayo Clinic EMR.

We demonstrated this capability in exhibits at the national Healthcare Information Management Systems Society (HIMSS) in New Orleans (2013) and Orlando (2014). When I retired, Mayo Clinic was using the software application suite to link into the partner organizations, and they were in the process of linking to the national network called eHealth Exchange at the time.

One of my last activities with the Consortium members was hosting a planning session at Mayo Clinic in Jacksonville for all of the team members working on the health information exchange. The focus of this planning session was to meet the clinical needs of the transplantation team at each of the provider sites for more information. There was general agreement by our respective physician staff members that if the clinical needs for the transplant physicians were satisfied with the quality of documentation provided, it would be sufficient for the other practice specialties.

The work of the Care Connectivity Consortium is in the best interest of all Americans. We were all proud to participate because health information exchange takes the efficiencies and benefits of the electronic medical record that we worked on for Mayo Clinic Jacksonville up to the national level, making a patient's information available at the point of care, wherever and whenever it is needed for the patient.

EPILOGUE

Retirement

The day started much as it normally did. I got up with the alarm at 5:15 a.m., pulled on my exercise clothes, shut off the burglar alarm, fixed a big mug of ice water, and took my first pill of the day. I wanted to have the ice water when I got off the recumbent bicycle after pedaling eight plus miles. I checked the coffeemaker for water, and then went to our exercise room. I adjusted the seat and started my half hour of daily aerobic exercise. I rode 8.1 miles while watching *Wake up with Al.*

With my exercise completed, I settled into my recliner in the family room and downloaded the morning newspaper on my iPad, so I could start reading before it actually arrived on the driveway a half hour or more later. At 6:15 I fixed my favorite, low-calorie breakfast. While things were warming in the toaster, I ran out to get the morning *Florida Times Union* paper and *The Wall Street Journal* from the driveway. When I returned, I had breakfast and coffee with the morning papers. I have followed this routine for years.

I dressed in my black suit, white shirt, and Hawaiian tie. I didn't know if anyone would notice it, but I anticipated being on vacation for the rest of my time at Mayo Clinic, officially retiring on July 1, 2014. I would complete twenty-four years of service to the day. The next two days I would be packing to leave for a three-week vacation in Hawaii, a perfect way to head into retirement.

The previous Sunday, I had cleared most of my things out of the office, and I planned to walk out of my office at the end of this day carrying just my briefcase, much like any other day. All of my personal things were already gone.

When I arrived, I logged into my Windows 7 workstation and my MacBook Air. I started Pandora, playing light classical music in the background. I used two computers: the MacBook, with the twenty-four-inch auxiliary screen, to run a WebEx meeting, and the PC to answer email or to draft documents. Nearly 175 email messages had accumulated since the previous day, with about 90 percent of them advertising IT products and services.

I had several remaining items that demanded my attention and resolution before I left for retirement. There was a trophy sitting on my shelf that had been there for nearly ten years, since December of 2005 to be precise. The inscription on the trophy read, "IT Florida 2005, Excellence in IT Leadership Northeast, Mayo Clinic."

The trophy was awarded to Mayo Clinic based on the work of the Applied Informatics Department, but my dilemma was how to handle it now that nearly a decade had elapsed. It was an awkward challenge. I drafted the story about the trophy and sent it to Dr. Mentel, proposing that I take it to the current CEO.

He agreed that it was the right thing to do. I printed the story, put it in a new folder, and walked over to the Davis Building, hoping to catch a few minutes with the CEO in Administration.

I found him and shared the story about the trophy. He seemed genuinely surprised and pleased to receive the trophy with the accompanying story. We walked over to the meeting room where other trophies were displayed and added it to the group. He opened the folder and placed the story under the trophy. He thanked me for my years of service and wished me well in retirement.

I grabbed a soft drink out of the cooler in the Coastal Room and walked out to the courtyard. I looked up at the clear blue sky and started my usual morning walk across campus. I typically took a walk to get away from my computers for a bit and to maintain my health.

Studies show a high correlation of spending more than two hours at a time in front of a computer with heart attacks. My walk was close to a mile, and springtime in Florida is beautiful. This day was no exception, and I reflected on my career with Mayo Clinic as I strolled across campus to the Cannaday Building. I thought about how the campus had grown and changed over the past twenty-four years.

Back in my office, I worked on a remaining draft for the new enterprise chief information officer. I was outlining the strategy for the Care Connectivity Consortium for near-term, intermediate-term, and long-term. At 11:20 I called James Houck. We had lunch plans in Jacksonville Beach.

That afternoon I finalized my draft for the CIO and sent it off. I walked over to Cannaday to say farewell to my good friend and colleague Dr. John Mentel. We visited for a while, and he again expressed his envy over my retirement, beating him to retirement *and* spending three weeks in Hawaii to celebrate.

I left his office and started back towards the hospital. My plan was to return to my office, and then go up to the second floor of the Stabile South Building, which housed most of the IT staff I had worked with over the years, and say farewell to some colleagues.

I debated about going by Administration to say good-bye to the current chair of administration. As I mulled it over while walking, I decided to drop by to speak with him, knowing he might not be available. If that were the case, I decided, "So be it!"

But he was available. I repeated the story I had told the CEO that morning, and he immediately wanted to see the trophy. We walked over to Administration, and I saw the CEO and an old friend of mine engaged in a conversation. I knocked on the door and asked to interrupt.

The old friend was Neal Patterson, the CEO and chair of the board for Cerner Corporation. Neal and I had worked together since 1992, when Dr. Black was the CEO and chair of the Board of Governors. I told Neal it was my last day at work for Mayo Clinic and I was heading to Hawaii soon.

I was very pleased that I had run into him on my last day. He congratulated me on my retirement, commented on how much he had enjoyed working with me over the years, and wished me all the best for the future. We shook hands, and I stepped out of the room and completed my conversation with the chair of Administration.

Walking back to Stabile South, I was energized by my good fortune. I spent time walking around to offices and cubicles, saying good-bye to people I had worked with over the years. I hired many of them during the time I was CIO for Mayo Clinic Jacksonville.

Upon returning to my office, I called Dr. Mentel. I thought he would find it interesting that Neal Patterson was back on campus and meeting with the CEO. We agreed to keep in touch after retirement. I shut off my workstation, picked up my briefcase, and walked out of my office into the warm spring sunshine.

On the way to the car, I reflected on the great individuals I had been blessed to work with over the years.

Dr. Leo F. Black was a visionary, brilliant with his absolute unflinching support he gave our team in working to automate the clinical practice.

My original physician partner brought his intelligence, wealth of clinical knowledge, and strong leadership throughout the formative days of the automation of the practice. He played a pivotal role in working with the physicians on so many of the automation issues.

The work he did on standardization of the structure of clinical notes was superb and continues to benefit the practice.

Dr. John Mentel brought such professionalism and so many computer skills that he was a strong advocate with technologists in making the hardware and software work to meet the needs of the physician users.

As I got into my car, I was grateful for all of the opportunities presented by the members of the staff, at all levels at Mayo Clinic.

APPENDIX

Observations

To do good is noble. To tell others to do good is even nobler and much less trouble.

—Mark Twain

I was blessed to have a career centered on systems, their development, and operations. This is a compilation of meaningful observations learned from those experiences. They are intended to benefit those who may find themselves inheriting some of the work and systems described here. Others may find challenges in understanding information technology and the potential to influence their healthcare operations. If any of these observations can help you avoid some expensive or painful learning, then it will have been worth it to include them here.

Application Programmers

Computer programmers love to build applications that are full of options through drop-down lists…in short, all kinds of "bells and whistles," as one of our physicians called it. Clinicians view too many options as time wasters. Simplify by reducing the number of mouse clicks and keyboard entries. Use defaults that reflect the clinician's most common choices but can be changed with a mouse click if necessary. Application programmers need to don white coats and shadow their clinical users for a day to see how their applications are being used in the clinical setting.

Change

Change is the enemy of stability. You will have to change to grow the system, update it, maintain it, and introduce new improved application software and databases for new organizational economies. Learn to install successive waves of change in technology with mastery. It is critical to keep the technology up-to-date and to achieve the optimal economies for your organization.

Clarity of Vision

When working on a project that has the potential to be transformational, all of the members need to be clear on the objective. Automation of the clinical practice can be ambiguous. We knew we had succeeded when we no longer needed to circulate the paper medical record to our physicians. It was a clear way to know our efforts had been successful.

Clinical Documentation

Nobody aspires to a health care profession because he or she loves to write clinical documentation. Expecting a physician to type his or her own clinical notes is not a good use of a physician's time. Strive to make the creation of clinical notes as easy and efficient as possible.

Continuous Quality Improvement

Continuous quality improvement is an effective way to improve quality and reduce waste in processes; however, it must permeate the organization's way of conducting business across the enterprise, from the CEO to the rank-and-file employee. Too often it is viewed as a project and becomes a "one-of," and then the organization moves on to selecting another quality project in another area. If the program isn't continuous, entropy ensues in the completed project area. In my professional career, I have witnessed continuous quality improvement (CQI) programs initiated into the operation of the same enterprise three or more times over a decade.

Effective Learning

No one likes to make mistakes in front of other people. If someone is learning new computer technology, he or she needs to learn it in a private setting before using the technology in front of others.

Goal of Automation

If you are not automating to go paperless, then you are automating for the wrong reason. You may end up with dual record systems, with all of the problems they create, and you will drive up the costs for your organization.

Information Architectures

At the time of this writing, a selection process has been completed at Mayo Clinic with the process of all sites being on a single electronic medical record and the replacement of the revenue cycle system. These are significant changes to the organization, and not without the associated risks. It is good to have the affirmation that the direction towards the integration of the information architecture selected back in 1992 is the direction for information systems at the enterprise level now, more than twenty years after the decision was made in Mayo Clinic Jacksonville.

Integrated Multispecialty Practice

The large integrated multispecialty practice that is Mayo Clinic is a model of how efficient medical practice can be. Patients who have gone through the conventional health care process immediately understand the benefits of the integrated multispecialty practice. The challenge of maintaining the integration is the ongoing work between the physicians and administrative leadership.

Live Demonstrations with Computers

In doing live system demonstrations, never compliment the computer. The computer will hear you and think to itself, *I'll show you!*

Murphy's Law

Murphy's Law is absolutely true. In computer technology anything that can go wrong, will, and at the worst possible moment, and will do the greatest amount of harm.

Partnerships

Selection of the partner for the electronic medical record is a critical decision that the enterprise will be forced to live with for a very long time. Moving petabytes of information between one system and another successfully by changing systems is far from trivial. Be sure the working relationship is well developed before getting into finalizing the contract details. We used to say that a good contract, once executed should go into a drawer and stay there.

I use the term partner instead of vendor because ideally, you want the relationship to function as a partner relationship. For a true partnership to be successful, both parties in the relationship need to be better off because they are partners than either would be on their own. That is the hallmark of a good partnership.

Productivity Management Systems

Productivity systems, when well understood, can be very effective in managing allied health workloads and gauging their economies. The indicators must be driven by statistics gathered from automated systems, not by humans. If you plan to use manual collection and reporting of data for any analysis, then find another way to collect the indicators. Productivity reports by manually collected counts and statistics aren't worth the paper they're written on.

System Integrity

The integrity of a system is no better than the integrity of the people engaged in inputting data and maintaining the system.

Systems Priority

With few exceptions, the physician is the most expensive "resource" in health care. Systems engineers need to keep their primary focus on making the physician as productive as possible.

Teamwork

When the Care Connectivity Consortium began its work, all of the project managers held a variety of positions within their respective organizations. In putting us all together, titles became meaningless since we worked for different companies, many miles apart. We all shared a common vision and charge. We rolled up our sleeves and went to work as a team with a common goal. It was a great experience and emphasized the old adage, "There is no limit to the amount of good that can be accomplished if it doesn't matter who gets the credit."

Technical Solutions

If given a clear problem to solve, information technologists can arrive at a solution. The problems arise when less knowledgeable leaders begin to get involved and politics takes over. Typically, a technology decision made by politicians is the worst possible technical solution.

Unscheduled System Downtime

In planning for high availability, remember computer hardware is all electromechanical devices. They will fail—it is not a matter of if, but when. Prepare for the failure; determine what must be done to recover the records and restore the system operation as quickly as possible.

Value Systems

In working with a large Christian faith-based healthcare organization prior to my work at Mayo Clinic, I witnessed personnel and business decisions that seemed ruthless to me. I couldn't believe the kinds of decisions made could come from people in an organization that professed Christian values. It wasn't until after I had worked at Mayo Clinic for a year or more that I realized the value systems in use at Mayo Clinic were the same values from the upper Midwest that I had witnessed as a young man growing up in Michigan. It was an ah-ha moment for me when I realized the difference between the two entities were those core values. Ironically Mayo Clinic is nondenominational but treats its business affiliates and personnel far better by comparison.

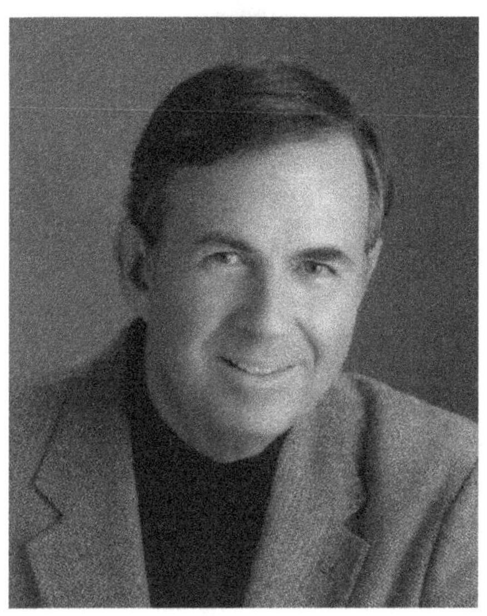

ABOUT THE AUTHOR

Reginald D. Smith is a native of Flint, Michigan. He holds a Bachelor of Arts from Andrews University, Berrien Springs, Michigan; a Master of Arts from the University of Michigan, Ann Arbor, Michigan; and the degree Doctor of Education from the University of Florida, Gainesville, Florida.

He retired from the Mayo Clinic Staff in 2014 with 24 years of service in Jacksonville and is now a member of the Emeritus Staff.

He lives with his wife of forty-eight years, Bonnie, on Lake Martin in east central Alabama.

www.ingramcontent.com/pod-product-compliance
Lightning Source LLC
Chambersburg PA
CBHW071730200326
41519CB00021BC/6646
9780998261805